THE KEYS⁑

A GUIDE TO A FLOURISHING LIFE

THE KEYS:

A Guide To A Flourishing Life

Ricardo M. Yslas

MILL CITY PRESS

Mill City Press, Inc.
2301 Lucien Way #415
Maitland, FL 32751
407.339.4217
www.millcitypress.net

Paperback ISBN-13: 978-1-66284-347-1
Hard Cover ISBN-13: 978-1-6628-4745-5
Ebook ISBN-13: 978-1-66284-348-8

SPECIAL THANKS

This book is dedicated to my Mom, Susan for revealing to me how to live in the light by showing me how one lives in the dark.

Thank you for your gifts.

Table of Contents

Note to Reader

It's been said that to know the light, we must know the dark and like all things there are two sides. We know one because of the other, we see and value one because of the other and each can help establish where we are and help guide us to where we want to be. Everyone defines success differently, yet there appears to be a collective agreement when asked what success is. Answers like:

- Independence (Physical and Financial)
- Health (Strength of Body, Mind and Spirit)
- Love (Familial and Romantic)
- Happiness (Unshakeable Well-being)

I believe these are all true and they are rooted in discipline. Success is a few simple disciplines practiced everyday. Disciplines build the foundation for those items above and keeps it solid. Even when we miss our mark, when we reflect back, try again, possibly this time in another way, we stay on the path of success. We keep our eye on the vision while seated at the table of life working our plan, planning the steps to get where we need to be, then we act on our plan. The only way we fail is if we stop on that path. A few errors in judgment repeated everyday without reflection or correction is how one fails. In this book, there are ten keys. Ten keys to the metaphorical locked doors keeping you from getting to where you want to go and who you want to be. My goal for this book is to educate through personal examples and those in history, as well as proven science to inspire the right action to help men and women flourish throughout the world.

Now, I'm no guru. I'm just a man and because of that I speak from experience and understanding with the information provided below. This isn't new material. No new truths. It's a rediscovery of what was there in the moment. It's from people who have lived and loved, lost and won. It's helped me and I believe it could help you. That's why I've organized it here. The researchers and philosophers, as well as other models of success spoken of will provide concrete examples of what is possible with these keys.

Now, I'll share with you some insights about who I am and provide a point of reference of where I come from so you and I may connect.

Unbeknownst to me the inspiration for this book began about 19 years ago when I was six years old. It wasn't until day in 2019 while reviewing old notes and reflecting, that I would be ready to assimilate the information I've gathered over the years. Going back now, I had been on Kent Island, Maryland, for three years. A small town where everyone knows just about everyone. Surrounded by water and the hospitality of the eastern shore, it was a heavenly place to have another beginning, more so than when we were living in Lanham, Maryland. Shortly after arriving on Kent Island, my brother was born. This is about the time I realized how different my parents were, my "coaches" in the way of the world at that time. My dad was the family leader, as are most dads and as we got older he became a source of wisdom for my brother and I. He involved us in as many activities as possible. Though I was a small kid growing up, I loved to be active in sports. At one time, my dad was afraid to sign me up for soccer because the smallest size shorts wouldn't fit.

Some of the most memorable sports we played were soccer, basketball, swimming, lacrosse and martial arts. We were also involved in Cub Scouts, Boy Scouts, Teen Court, and the Rocket Club. Outside of the sports arenas, my dad was always pushing for education. "Read and learn as much as possible" and "develop a vocabulary" were some of his greatest sayings. When my mom was around, she was a listening ear and an emotional support but that was few and far in between. When I was in 3rd grade she left for a rehab center. In middle school, she was arrested and put in jail for a year. Most of the lessons I learned from her came by way of the opposite and much reflection later. I got to see from her, how commitment, dedication, and relentlessness to the wrong things and people even when you want the best for yourself and your family isn't enough. As I was growing up I saw people just like her though who turned it around, using the same virtues but for a higher purpose. Seeing these new possibilities, I was convinced someone like her could excel in all arenas of life too, if she made that decision.

I was soon to understand though that addiction is devastating. It takes people with great potential, and maimes them; sometimes against their own will. It's more powerful than love yet research is finding a key to beating addiction in the chemistry of love we will discuss in a later chapter. Fast forward to age twelve, I had become rebellious; angry at the world for the hand I felt I had been dealt. Between fights in school, struggling with school work and the chaos of home life, I wanted to wage a war. Michael Holt illustrates this feeling in A Call To Arms:

> "In the embryonic stage of his radical development, he yearns only to fight. The state of things, his own search for truth, his lack of self understanding, these all combine to create the perfect storm of anger in his developing warrior heart. Initially, it is this anger that fuels this revolutionary's rebellion. His anger is projected upon the external power structures he feels has taken his autonomy and the autonomy of many. The fire in his angry heart burns brighter and brighter…"

Hearing fights and arguments between my parents and even being the subject of many fights on the way to sports practice, my love for each of my parents had me pulled in two directions. This was the same year I was brought along, for the first time, on a drug deal with my mom and witnessing her doped up friends. This shook me. I turned to other means of coping and started to drink when my parents weren't around. I was in 8th grade. In the same year is when I found inspiration in the members of the armed forces. I saw Rambo and Saving Private Ryan and though they were fictional films I was inspired by the story and began training daily. The pain of the workouts took my mind away from the pain of the circumstances in front of me. I could only focus on one. The burn of the exercises, then the calmness that followed after, had me coming back to training again and again. I thought if I could be like those men on the screen, have a mission and walk with a unit, my family would come together and join in this mentality. They didn't. At least not in the way I had envisioned.

Entering high school I found a mentor named Mr.L, a school computer teacher and powerlifting coach. After school, when swimming wasn't in season, this was dedicated gym time. School got out at 2:30 pm. I'd walk down the hall to the gym and I'd lift until I was told to go home. I'd leave all the frustrations of the day on the gym floor in the form of sweat. In 10th grade I got involved with some hooligans and dabbled into marijuana. I was 15 years old. Feeling lethargic and eating the wrong foods, seeing grades decline and even hearing about one of the dealers we know get his house raided twice, I stopped cold turkey. I remember being in my friends house after smoking and just being disgusted with the time and potential I was wasting- I got on the floor and began doing sit-ups to kill the high. I removed these friends from my day to day and dove deeper into studying nutrition, supplementation and methods of training. Now, this didn't play out as clean and effortless as it reads. I had deep depressions from lost relationships, some driving me to thoughts of taking my own life on three accounts. It wasn't until I met a young woman and her family that I found another purpose and got to see a cohesive family, one that I wasn't related to and I could participate in, that my mindset began to mature. I was able to put someone else before myself and also begin teaching what I was learning about in

health, exercise and dieting. I learned to listen in a new way as well as learn to be taught. I was learning how to love.

As sweet as that sounds, it ended 3 years later. Leaving with it adventure and a plethora of experience. After a major push from her father to start working, I got my first job at Abercrombie and Fitch then moved to Teavana, then to GNC.

Working for GNC at first seemed like a mistake. I shopped there for years before working there and it always seemed alive and engaging. Being an employee though, it was different. It was dead most days and just another guy and I worked in the store. Compared to being around models and constant customer traffic at Abercrombie and Teavana, this new environment and sales training was challenging. Here though, is where I learned about persuasion and sales, human nature, and learning to confront my own fears. And, later when managing my own store, how to reflect, journal, study and meditate. I found another mentor at GNC named Hunter. He was one of the best sales managers in the district and one of the youngest guys to make regional sales director in the company ever. Being around him and observing his routine, observing his sales techniques and habits and then seeing the results he achieved, I was inspired. Using the information from him and other mentors and engaging in activities like theirs from ages 19-21, I was learning to take myself where I wanted to go, mentally, emotionally and physically, by developing habits that would get me there. I stopped drinking and instead poured myself into training my mind and body daily. During this time with my trainer and mentor, Derek, I accomplished an elite level squat at 205 lbs body weight squatting 530 lbs with a bum knee. I was promoted at work for excellent sales, opening the first GNC on Kent Island and became its first manager. Things were looking good.

At age 22, having gathered some knowledge in health and fitness working for GNC, studying to be a personal trainer and training others, I began writing a book called The Peach: A Guide to a Better Booty, a book inspired by and for the positive women in my life. At this time working for GNC, I was still planning on enlisting in the military.

While working one day I met a trainer who led a program for military personnel looking to join the special forces. It was a program for enlisted men and US Naval Academy students. I was interested but I wasn't enlisted. With some influence and persuasion though, I got by the restriction and signed up for the training beginning in January of 2016. It was not what I anticipated. The training was great, the style and intensity I enjoy but the people in the program with the exception of two officers did not embody the values one thinks of when imagining someone in uniform. After being lied to and finding out about an infidelity between one of my team members best friends and my romantic partner, I dropped the program.

After deciding that's not the group I'd want to work alongside, I went back to my roots in 2016 and began training for an MMA fight. I realized that even though I wasn't joining the military anymore I could still embody military values and use them in my life. Again burning my pain as fuel, training kept me focused. My training partner at the time was an aggressive wrestler. Tough as nails and strong. We would exchange several heavy blows in a round, some of which earned me my first concussion. We called off the fight shortly after. I noticed that burning my pain as fuel was getting me injured more than it was growing my body, mind and spirit. The dark energy got me in the game, got me started but I realized it was the light that sustained me when things were getting tougher.

> *"...Inevitably, he learns the lesson that all who use anger to fuel their rebellion must learn: he learns he has burned himself with his own flame."*

In December of 2016, I graduated from Chesapeake College with a Liberal Arts of Science degree. At the beginning of 2017 I left GNC and started a new job doing telecommunications work for my cousin and uncle that required that I get up at 3:00 am, five days a week involving physical labor. Two weeks into it, I was stirred up with the people I was partnered with and exhausted after work, falling asleep at the wheel most days and passing out in the driveway when I got home. Still writing The Peach, I had almost no time to work on it. I could hardly think, it was killing my creativity so I called my boss, my cousin, and expressed this. I wanted out of this job and to go back to school. Leaving though, I let my uncle down as well as myself. I missed the deadline to enroll for school and now had all day to write. In two 8-hour sessions I finished the third chapter on nutrition. Two weeks later while at the community college library writing, my uncle called and we talked about what happened and what I needed to do. I still remember his words: "You're earning good money. Money gives you options. I'm giving you options." And knowing my love of training and my inspiration from the military, he said: "you think you would just leave boot camp because it's tough, because you're tired? Would you leave the field?"

I came back to this job. This time determined and with a plan. A financial plan, a health plan and with the resolve to learn the skills needed to excel everyone where I worked. Nothing and no one would stop me. I finished the final chapter that spring, writing at night before bed and in the van on the way to jobs sites. I wasn't welcomed back either by the other guys. I was now known and mocked as "the creative one". It took almost 6 months before we got along. Now, two years later, I still hear about it but now in a more playful way.

As I healed up and moved through the first concussion, I trained regularly as well as coached twice a week until getting rhabdomyolysis from a 16 mile run and earning another concussion from a sparring match in Bowie, November of 2017. The only difference this time was that I knew how to handle it. Again recovering from the second concussion from sparring, and working a telecommunications job, there was just work and the kind I wasn't interested in, nor did I see eye to eye with a majority of the people I worked with. I hadn't yet earned their trust and respect. I took time to reflect and account of where I was, where I really wanted to be and who as person I needed to become to just be. I reflected on the skills as well as financial numbers I needed to reach to obtain what I valued. I realized I needed to turn what I have developed inside and start bringing it outward to those available from a place of groundedness.

Coming into the new year and still being the newest and youngest guy on this team, I needed to build trust and earn respect in the field. I found another mentor named Kris, a seasoned manager, to guide me in how to bend conduit, install cable trays and read blueprints. I had a meeting with him and asked to take on a small job on the third floor of the hospital installing cable tray, pulling in the cable and terminating the drops. I got the green light in October to perform these tasks, and got to work finishing everything by December of 2017.

Training regularly, reading and writing were taken away for a moment that seemed to stretch into eternity at the end of that year and into 2018. By July 2018, I began to feel myself regaining my sharpness in mind and body. In that period between November and July though, this experience made clear to me that everything is transient. I realized as tough as one may get, as smart as one may be, it can and will be taken from you at some point. Amidst my brain fog, my priorities and values became very clear. I made a list of things to protect including my mind, my sleep, my diet, and money, why these were important and how to better use them. I realized, if I am to make an impact in my life and those around me, and be remembered, I must begin working on building a legacy. I was reminded, our time here is only for a little while.

Over a year has passed since the injuries, and with it, friends and mentors have come and gone. Many stories have been shared and deeper bonds between my family, friends and coworkers have formed. I wouldn't change any of it. Each has taught me a lesson in its time when I became aware of what I was doing and aided me in getting clear on what results I wanted. I'm reminded of two quotes. The first is by the American Tibetan Buddhist Pema Chödrön: "Nothing ever goes away until it has taught us what we need to know."[2] and the second and a yoga practitioner: "If there is a negative habit, addiction, or problem that keeps repeatedly showing up in your life, know that it holds a deep message for you."[3]

Again this reads clean on paper. Many conversations unheard behind closed doors, long drives, moments of intense joy and love as well as dark dreary days have ascertained their rhythms in between these lines, allowing the moment I have now to unfold. The people around us, our family and community are what make our triumphs worth our sacrifices and our losses less burdensome.

The point I'm making is this:

It's less about who we are, where we are and what we can do and more about what you will do and how you can make those around you do well. It's how you frame it. One bad chapter doesn't define the book. Though we cannot write a new beginning, we can write a new ending. Even if you're six years old and your shorts don't fit, sign up, show up. Even if your mom or dad isn't all you need them to be, there's always someone doing well you can reach out to at school, at the gym, or in the neighborhood. If things aren't the way you want them to be, you have the power to change that. Books are available, videos are available. When your program fails or your plan flops, it's only a lesson learned, it's an opportunity to pivot, keep the same drive and energy and go in a new direction. My brief story above is only an example of what many others experience as well but may not speak of. We all have ups and we all have downs. We must remember the darkness is not a home, it's a tool. You cannot live there and live a flourishing life, you have to use it. The difference I want you to see is that if you want more wins in your life, be willing to get back up and go again and again and again, into your fire, into your mind, into your place of work until you're done, until you win. I want to help you. Your success is critical to my success. As we walk this path of the ten keys together, know that I'm rooting for you and I'm greatly looking forward to your growth and development.

> *": When the fire of anger dies and gives way to*
> *the fire of love - the sky blazes."*

Here's an overview of each chapter and what we will cover.

In chapter one we will cover Story. How identification affects our emotions and how to structure our identity so as to feel the way we need for mission success. We will discuss how repetition, emotion and consistency build a healthy self image and destroy old paradigms as well define belief and where it is in our body.

In chapter two we define then learn to objectively see our habits, how they affect us and how to build new ones through practice and how the seemingly insignificant affects the monumental outcomes of our daily lives. We will be finding direction through determining our philosophy, and how to know if you are on the right path. Then we explore Love, where it originates, it's effects on us as well as others, its ability to heal through the hormone oxytocin and how to create more love in our lives.

Our focus in chapter three is on Models and the traits they embody. We will discuss how to go about finding a model, when it's time to leave our model and strike out on our own path.

Chapter four is on influence. We will define our current circle of influence and learn to become aware of the ways in which they have power in our lives. We will find how influence affects you and how you affect others with it. We will also discuss the ways in which body language affects our ability to influence.

In chapter five we dive into the science of leadership and human connection. We will find what stress is and its effects short term and long term, what parts of the brain this stems from and how to better use that stress. We will peer into how those at the top think, their responsibility, their reward and consequences.

In chapter six we will learn how to identify our gifts and abilities and how we can leverage those gifts and abilities to heal others and provide support where needed.

Chapter seven is on Mastery. We will find out how to use process to build consistent wins in our lives, as well as the power of the beginning and end of our day. We will discover how practical thinking combined with our dreams become reality and how to repeat the process in other areas of our lives. We will find how self mastery is the greatest freedom and the two types of freedom available to us. Lastly we learn how to set a system in place to achieve the goals we set for ourselves.

Chapter eight is on Sabbath, rest, recovery and learning to slow down our mind and body so as to give our body, mind and spirit an opportunity to grow.

Chapter nine is on Friendship. The importance of proper friends, how friends form, the effects of good and bad friends and how to come together with people of differences, put them aside and complete a common objective.

Chapter ten is on Death and coming to understand it. We will discuss how it provides a sense of value to our days and come to use our knowledge of our mortality with urgency to, not only check the boxes we have on our lists, but how it's free us to live authentically.

In the conclusion of this book I include a list of characteristics from what I strive to emulate and those of great achievement had and have, called "What A Man Is" and "Ways to Be Your Best Self". Though the first one is geared toward men, the characteristics are universal. I can only speak from one side though. I'd love to hear from you ladies what you believe makes a Woman and the rites of passage for young ladies.

May the keys here unlock your potential and open the doors of possibility for you and those around you.

Chapter 1:

Story: A Quest

"Who do you want to be?
Not what, but who?" [7]
—Arnold Schwarzenegger

OF ALL THE many ways there are to think, we most often think in stories. The human mind is narrative. How did we get the idea of who we are today and what's possible for us as well as others? We were told stories. We learn who we are, where we come from, right and wrong, morals and values from hearing and telling stories.

It's something we have heard from the time we were born and will continue to hear throughout our lives. The problem with most stories though, is they seem just that, stories made up and unlikely to happen to the person hearing them. A message only resonates when it touches a part of your life you have known and experienced but it can provide a concept before experience happens.

For children, having very limited experiences of the world, hearing stories of three piggies finding the proper home or a wicked stepmother or a wooden boy whose nose grows when not telling the truth gives them a concept of the way the world is and the consequences of it. Deprive children of these stories and we leave them unscripted, without simple models to guide their words and conduct their actions. When we claim an identity or identify with a character, we also claim the commitments and values these characters embody.

The characters in the stories we read and illustrations we see and in the latest century, movies, set the stage for children. As adults though, it's often forgotten that instead of just listening to stories of the past, hearing them retold, we have the power to rescript our narrative. We have the power to write history in the way we choose, even when the odds are against us. Viktor Frankl, a prisoner in Auschwitz during World War II, is a prime example of this:

> *"Everything can be taken from a man but one thing: the last of the human freedoms— to choose one's attitude in any given set of circumstances, to choose one's own way."*[8]

If you're reading this though, it's highly likely you've lived beyond your elementary years and have formed a story of who you are, where you come from and what's possible for you based on circumstances, past and current.

You may be satisfied with right now. That's great. Carry on. Life will change though. Life is always oscillating and the tables do turn and how you handle that rotation will determine your level of respect and love for yourself as well as the character you develop and the relationships you form.

As with Viktor Frankl, you and I are meeting in what literature calls "in medias res" or in the middle of things. We meet Dr. Frankl long after he has become a doctor, survived the treacherous concentration camps and written his books. I am meeting you after 25 years of treading upon the earth and I meet you where you are now after a journey from where you have come from. For some, that has been the street over, or it may have been on a train in California or on a bus in Ireland. Either way, at that moment, no matter what has come before, the story begins in the present moment, our story begins now. Time in our stories ebbs and flows from past to now, from now to the future, back to now. May this moment be one of the best to come.

> Live as if you were living a second time, and as
> though you had acted wrongly the first time.
> —Viktor Frankl

Our lives aren't just one story either. We play many roles upon the places we go. Your story will contain elements of triumph and defeat, love and loss, life and death, rivalry and revenge, sacrifice and indulgence and not just one time but many times. In these repetitions, our story is being written and our character developed. Another way to think of this is in terms of a quest. Joseph Campbell's book *The Hero with a Thousand Faces* tells of such a tale. In his book, Campbell uses a plethora of heroes from different eras and cultures. Campbell believes a "hero" isn't a perfect person who always gets things right. A hero is someone who "found or achieved something beyond the normal range of achievement and who has given his life to something bigger than himself or other than himself."[9] In this way, by going on a journey, we find out about the true nature of what it is we desire in life, that job, that status, that relationship.

In these stories the hero is "called". To be called has its roots in religion: it means being called by God. Many of you may know this feeling of being pulled toward a particular kind of work, even when the odds seem stacked against you or the task itself is difficult. I felt this when writing my first book. It had to be done. This work works on you as much as you work on it, over time becoming pleasurable as we learn to maneuver in that space and handle the hardship that comes with it.

Our calling is an echo of our efforts in life and the ripples of others in our environment. After the call, the hero is led down a road of trials and tribulations, successes and failures. As they travel this path, they meet people that assist them along the way. People seasoned and experienced in the endeavor the hero is passing through. The hero, when humble, learns from those not as far along on their path as they are. These experienced people often serve as mentors and those less experienced allow the hero to set an example. Allies and enemies are formed and battles are fought. In fighting, losing and winning, the hero learns how to fight, when to fight and when to throttle back. Relationships are lost and some rekindled and some newly formed. On this journey, the hero overcomes their fear of combat with others by engaging with them often and with that comes "special powers" or skills and they find gifts in the form of advice from those they encounter. As they trek on this path, they continue to meet triumph and defeat but succeeding more than they fail, continually growing stronger and more resilient over time while they strive for their potential, meeting more challenges and triumphs.

The hero, sometimes before or after beginning their journey, is faced with what Campbell calls an "abyss" meaning, a large failure. This failure is a test to see if the hero has the strength, resilience and determination to face the obstacle again, this time from a new position, a new mindset. If they continue to push forward they undergo a change or metamorphosis, becoming witness to their own fears and deficiencies without losing their drive and ambition that continues to thrust them forward.

They learn calculated fearlessness. Becoming strategic and wise. Knowing what poses a real threat and what can be brushed aside. With all the battles the hero faces and all the triumphs as well as defeats they experience, the greatest gift they receive is what Campbell calls the "boon" meaning knowledge of how to succeed in that particular arena. This carries on for many years. As time passes, more successes and more rewards are accumulated, becoming less and less thrilling and fulfilling. What fulfills the hero now is passing on this knowledge to those in their circle, what Campbell calls "returning the boon." You may notice this in many grandparents, widely traveled people and even younger men and women who are doing well after facing defeats and overcoming them. Once the boon is returned, the hero is free to savor life until death takes them on another journey.

> "...Character, as thus defined, is developed
> through contests with tough adversaries,
> through wrestling with real problems, through
> mastering difficult situations."[10]
> —Basic Principles of Speech

Most of us have heard, "Don't be a hero." or "I'm no hero." And in many cases that's true. You will have the fecal matter kicked out of you, you will be berated with comments and attacks, a lot of times from people you care about and admire most. It's hard work, yet rewarding in a way few people understand. Those that do understand though, can make sense of why others would want to partake on that path. Let's talk about how we find our character. This leads us into three-steps:

- Identify

- Act
- Feel

To dig into the past for you may be too much to bear right now and if it is, I understand. Those willing to do this work though will reap a bounty. It's been found that people with a sense of their past and their family history are usually better able to manage hardships in the present because being part of a story, we're no longer alone. Seeing what others have done, we come to understand more fully our responsibility to ourselves and other members of our community.

In the steps above, many people mix the order up and use feeling first, then action then identification. It looks rational and is easy to follow but will lead to a downward spiral when the hot gates of adversity open or when sweet bliss enters our lives. Feelings are important, they are also often misguided and not based on fact, on reality. They do not last very long. A few seconds to a few minutes if fully felt. Moods are different and can drag into hours or even days. Let's talk about that for a moment.

A commonly asked question when someone is under the weather is to ask: "What are you feeling?"

The objective of this question is to find out what action you should take. The problem though is that feelings are fickle. Just because you don't feel like it, doesn't change the fact that the task you need done is still waiting to be engaged and finished. It doesn't change our responsibility to ourselves and those around us. Even more important, the more you act on feelings, the more it becomes a habit and over time, that's who you become.

> If the kids are crying, if you don't feel like it, if
> your back hurts, if you've got aches and pains...
> It's still your motherf*cking set. Get it done![12]
> —CT Fletcher

Better questions to ask are:

- "Who do you want to become?"
- "Who do you want to be?"

With these questions we are able to create or find a model, a virtue or principle that goes unchanging that can be our rod and staff when faced with difficulty. We have an azimuth to guide us into action, which in turn will lead to feelings. One of the things I was taught in theater while in college was that the faces you make, the clothing you wear, the behavior you take on will create feelings. Just by breathing shallowly and furrowing your brow, you will feel anxious or angry and those types of thoughts will surface. You've stimulated the sympathetic nervous system. On the other hand, if you take long deep breaths, relax your body, your mind will relax, thoughts may cease or be pleasant. You've stimulated the parasympathetic nervous system. In short, if you want to feel differently, act differently. **Our mind is rooted in our physiology.**

With identity first, we knowingly choose to be a particular type of person. How we see the world around us changing, and how we view success changes too. Because at our core level, our character is altered by identifying first with who we want to be. There are certain actions that lead to positive consequences. We see certain characters win. Just because you're talented or gifted in a certain field doesn't make you a good person, or a successful person. It simply shows you are competent, which is nonetheless important but alone competence is not enough to live a flourishing life. You have to have the character that goes with it. Character precedes talent everyday of the week. One of the best definitions of Character I've found is in the book *Basic Principles of Speech* by Sarett Foster: Character is "the sum of the attributes of a man's mind, of his body, of his heart and his spirit." While we cannot promise we will reach our goal, we can forge the character worthy of that achievement.

> Set the kind of goals that will make something of
> you to achieve them.
> —Jim Rohn

For those feeling types out there, feelings are significant, not just for developing character but for forming relationships. One in particular, is empathy. Empathy is the ability to understand and share the feelings of another. A disciple once asked Confucius, "Is there a single word that can be a guide to conduct one's life?" Confucius said "It is perhaps the word empathy."[13]

Another great analogy of emotions comes from the Ancient Greek philosopher Plato in his vision of the tri-partite nature of the soul. Plato uses a chariot pulled by two horses as an example in his dialogue, *Phaedrus*. The chariot is pulled by two winged-horses, one mortal and the other immortal. The mortal horse is described as "a crooked heavy ill put together animal of a dark color with grey bloodshot eyes; the mate of insolence and pride, shag-eared and deaf, hardly yielding to whip and spur."[14] This is our appetites and baser emotions. In modern terms stemming from our reptilian portion of our triune brain. The immortal horse, similar to the mammalian part of the brain, is described as upright and cleany, carrying his neck high. He has an aqui-line nose and his color is white. His eyes dark. He is a lover of honor and modesty and temperance, and the follower of true glory; he needs no touch of the whip, but is guided by word and admonition only." Then there is the charioteer who guides the two horses. The charioteer represents our reason, stemming from our neocortex, the newest addition of our brains.

Where does this charioteer fly? The ridge of heaven, where it may encounter the Nature of the Divine: Beauty, Goodness, Justice, Knowledge, Truth and Wisdom. These elements nourish the wings of the horses, keeping them healthy, keeping the chariot in flight. A charioteer flys with the gods and is led by Zeus on this flight into heaven. The difference between the gods' chariot and a mortal soul's chariot is that the gods have two immortal horses pulling them, making their flight effortless. Man has one mortal horse though, making conditions ripe for turbulence and struggle. The white horse wishes to rise while the dark horse pulls the chariot down towards the earth away from the heavens. As each horse battles to lead, the charioteer has to get them working together on a single purpose, ideally rising into the heavens. With this duo, they ride close to the ridge of the heavens, catching a momentary view of it before falling below the surface, rising then falling again, like waves rolling along the shore.

If the charioteer is able to view these forms, he is able to continue flying with the gods around heaven. If he cannot pilot his chariot and control his horses, the horses' wings will wither from lack of nourishment or become destroyed through vices of vileness and evil, from battling one another. In the latter case, the chariot will plummet to earth, the horses lose their wings and the human soul is manifested in the flesh. Depending on fall and the rank of the mortal body the soul has taken up, the length of time it takes for the horses to regrow their wings will vary. The life of this body may be one of a philosopher, an artist, a king, a tyrant, or politician or some other worldly character. Whoever was more justly while guiding the chariot gets the better lot on earth. In short, the more truth discovered on the ridge of heaven, the shallower the fall and the better life the soul leads. Encounters with people that contain essences of divinity, reminding him or her of their past existence, increase the speed at which the wings of their horses grow as well, thus allowing the soul to return to heaven more quickly.

In Plato's allegory we see three things. Both horses are needed to pull the chariot upward, our emotions are something separate from us and when both our emotions and our reason are in sync, one obtains harmony.

We cannot let logic dominate our day to day lives just as we cannot allow emotions to rule our decision making. It's okay to *feel* jealousy, anger, injustice and greed. That's normal, that's part of the human experience. With training and consistent practice, those vices can be transcended into virtues. It's energy is transferred into actions that further "grow our wings", your ability to help yourself and help others win. It's not okay though, to *be* jealous, angry, injust, or greedy. **The objective is to tame our desires.** Whether it's a want for a particular food, particular person, or particular item. There is no difference. Being disciplined, but knowing what you want, what you desire will determine your course of action and if you really need it to flourish. I believe a toilet paper company said it well: "less is more".

Focus on the process knowing first what you want. You'll get what you focus on because we see only that which we aim at. Hone this power. Keep it close and never give it away. If you want more, work in a way that's going to produce well-being, strength, abundance and knowledge. Just as important, be patient. Learn to be here in this moment, after having set the plans in action for the future. Both are necessary and need to be revisited often.

When you move, move deliberately, with initiative and strength. Power will develop. This is what it means to know your course just like the charioteer flying around heaven. Use your internal compass. Adjust as needed, yet stay true to your nature and your end goal. Again the objective is to tame our desires, not remove them. Channel and transcend the desire into its highest virtue. Great things happen that way and they last longer. They echo for generations and in generations. Otherwise, you will fall like the souls in Plato's dialogue who could not maintain the look upon the Divine, having to work a lifetime to glimpse at Heavens which are here on earth with us now.

> I have learned through bitter experience the one
> supreme lesson to conserve my anger, and as heat
> conserved is transmuted into energy, even so our
> anger controlled can be transmuted into a power
> which can move the world.[15]
> —Gandhi

Some other questions we ask others are:

Why do you feel that way?

What makes you feel that way?

When did you start to feel this way?

Who have you talked to about this?

Where do you feel like this most often?

The question that carries the most weight though is asking how. "How do you make yourself feel that way?" To someone doing well, we rarely ask any questions of why, what, when, who or where. We just accept it until we want a part of the harvest. Then we want to know how. This question of how can seem rude and uncaring to someone hurting, yet when we fail to ask it, three things happen.

One, we fail to identify and come to understand a deeper source of the feelings. Two, without challenge there can be no triumph, no victory. In fact, challenging someone, in a way that is helpful to their development is a sign of respect. Certain feelings and emotions, like those evoked from death and major loss are to be mourned, are to be embraced. If not embraced and felt fully, they linger and can cause psychological disorder later. It's when emotions and habits begin to negatively affect our life and that of others counting on us that a challenge is needed to lift us above our immediate suffering. And three, we fail to give this person an opportunity to take the reins of their situation, to gain control of themselves.

One way I personally change my negative feelings or enhance my positive feelings is by going to the gym or just exercising in general. As a kid I discovered this effect and used it to propel myself through many chaotic moments growing up. It became part of my identity and is part of my identity today. I don't just lift weights, I am a lifter. I don't just swim, I'm a swimmer. I am aware that the gym is not an atmosphere for everyone but exercising is a way to take control of oneself and that feeling of control brings confidence and security to other areas of one's life. They may not be a "gym person" but they likely know exercise is healthy and we all want to be healthy. We all want to be able to do more for ourselves. Training our body allows that to happen. If someone you know isn't making changes, it's likely they identify as being someone unrelated to their goal. Someone who just does the motions lacking the energy behind the movement. That's half the equation missing and with only half, we miss our whole, our being, our character. The labels we give ourselves and objects matter. **The small things are the big things.**

Related to exercise, someone may have had a bad experience and have fallen off course. Understandable. If they performed at a pace and intensity relative to their ability though, they may have found it pleasurable and confidence building, allowing that behavior to more than likely stick and over time change their physiology, their mindset and their sense of self. It doesn't take radical change to make meaningful progress. It doesn't take much to feel good about yourself. One rep. One step is a start. Just keep repping and stepping and your identity will change. One workout complete, you're an athlete. One book read, you're a reader. One class done, you're a student. One dollar saved, you're a saver. One dollar invested, you're an investor. This could happen over a matter of hours. The key is doing it again and again and again. Sixty-six consecutive days on average says the University College London is how long it takes to form a new habit at a minimum.[17] Being that habits form our identity, that's how long on average it will take you to <u>begin</u> to feel this new you.

As mentioned earlier, our psyche is rooted in our physiology. Sometimes referred to as our mind-body connection. Moving our body, we literally take our stagnant, blocked energy and move it, transforming it into its opposite energy, vitality and vigor. Jumping, running, lifting heavy, throwing a ball or hitting a mitt or bag provides an outlet to channel emotions into. We perform certain emotions by the way we move our bodies and through our posture. Look at where your energy is going. This means your attention and more specifically your body. Where is your mind taking your body?

Energy + Motion = Emotion

As an example of physiology affecting moods, the psychologist Dr. David Burns has an extreme example of how well exercise can turn a negative emotion into a positive one.

Here is a report of one of his videos recorded sessions with a patient having a panic attack:

The patient looks around frantically. She is sobbing, panicking, overwhelmed by anxiety. She says she can't breathe; her lungs are about to collapse; her heart is about to stop. She feels like she is going to die.

Listening to this, David D. Burns calmly asks her, "Do you think you could exercise strenuously right now?" Terri doesn't know; she just feels so bad. "Why don't we find out?" Burns suggests. "What's the most strenuous exercise you could do? Jumping jacks? Running in place?"

Terri says "I feel dumb" as she runs in place. "That's okay," Burns says. "If you have to feel dumb to get well, it would be worth it." Terri says she feels dizzy. "OK, well just keep going," Burns says, and then asks her to try some jumping jacks.

"Could you do this if you were dying?" he asks Terri. "Can you see yourself in an emergency room doing jumping jacks?" Hesitantly, she begins to laugh. Soon she's belly laughing. The joy she feels surges off the screen. Turning from the video to the therapists, Burns says that's the kind of dramatic change he wants them to achieve. Terri had been experiencing five paralyzing panic attacks a week. She's had only one since Burns taped the session they've just viewed—and that was 20 years ago.

Though this is an extreme example it applies to us as humans. With the proper knowledge, some encouragement and a little bit of chutzpah, we can turn a moment of intense fear into an enjoyable experience or at minimum, better bear our pain. At the end of his video training, Dr. David Burns addresses a key insight to the other therapists viewing this recording. The pain and anxiety this woman experienced may be specific to her, but it is not unique. That feeling bears a likeness to losing a job as the breadwinner and not knowing where your next meal will come from or even a break up and separation from a loved one. The key is to find out how others in our community, others in history have succeeded and overcome their pain. Someone, somewhere has experienced this feeling and transcended it. Seek them out and learn their way, then shape it to your circumstances.

From the example above, notice she didn't do just one jumping jack or just one exercise. She tried a couple exercises, she did repetitions _until_ she felt better. As in the gym, one repetition is to find maximums and test our strength but that way of training is a poor stimulus for developing resilience in the face of pain and the ability to endure the hardship that comes when developing new habits, identity and character. Some things in life need only to be done once. They can be marked as finished. We can check the box and move to our next thing, never to return to that item again. Like good hygiene though, shaping our body, mind and spirit is daily work. Some days are easy, we move fluidly, we absorb our environment with keen senses and our spirit is cheerful. Other days are long, dark, cold and wear our spirits down. But when we practice daily, taking in a visual and physical diet of good food and good exercise, we build our body, our belief and confidence to withstand negative forces and strengthen our resolve to design the best version of ourselves. The struggles we face are necessary to form our sense of who we are and what we are capable of. It is attempting to summon us to show up, be stronger and forge an identity that's vital to a flourishing life. Through repetitions of work, training, and love, we forge a new identity.

Now some of you may be wondering:
"Where do I begin?"

It begins with your belief. It begins by believing. Believing in yourself that you can become that Man, become that Woman, that identity. **What is a belief? A belief is a group of cells that have been connected and reinforced.** Put another way, neurons that fire together wire together. By repeating certain actions, we create habits, we develop neural maps of how to operate. We form an idea of who we are. We plant a seed if you will. As these neurons continue to fire together they connect with more and more synapses creating a deeper and deeper belief, a vast interconnectedness that weaves itself into all areas of our lives. Because of this design in our physiology, even a thing that is false can become a reality for us. The same is for good habits and bad habits. The more we hear something, the more we perform a task, the less we have to consciously use our will to summon that energy, the less we notice it and we come to "be" that way and we then identify with that, which is what people call our character. Our character can be cultivated through our consciousness, through our awareness. **The character we embody will determine where we go, what we do and how we feel, thus determining our results.**

> The chains of habit are too light to be felt
> until they are too heavy to be broken.[19]—
> Warren Buffett

The longer we wait, the harder and more difficult it is to change who we are because of our mental maps. Just because it's hard though, doesn't mean you shouldn't go for it. Don't wait another day. So just like wealth and skills, strength and love, character and identity, our lives are not built by one moment, one dramatic act, but by accumulation, by small unspectacular decisions made every day.

Before we leave this chapter I'd like to leave you with a story containing elements of what we discussed in this chapter. This is the Story of the Sower.[20]

The Story of the Sower

The sower was ambitious.
He had excellent seed.

The sower goes out to sow the seed, but the first part of the seed falls by the wayside and the birds get it.

The birds are going to get some of the seed.
If you go chasing birds, you leave the field. These birds are people who pick at you or who withdraw from your life.

Chasing them distracts from your future, rather than adding to it.

The sower keeps on sowing. If you keep on sowing, there isn't enough for the birds to eat.

The rocky ground where the soil is shallow kills off some of the seeds. That's okay, it's not of your making. This is our circumstances. But because you are an ambitious sower and have excellent seed, you keep on sowing.

Some seeds begin to sprout in the shallow ground until the sun comes up.
The hot day will wither some of your plants.
Let it be. Say "That's interesting." and sow again.
It's wise to learn to discipline your disappointment.
Meaning mourn, then move forward. It's now fuel and part of the story, your story.

The seed falls on thorny ground. The plants begin to grow again. The thorns choke the plants and they die. Thorns are going to get some.

These thorns are little distractions.

People let little things cheat them out of big opportunities. Focus on your harvest, yet stay aware of pitfalls.

Do the little things that count. Look past the little things that don't. See the final scene of what you are seeking to achieve, who you are seeking to become.

The sower keeps on sowing the seed.
He keeps taking action.

Finally, the seed falls on good ground. It always will if you keep sowing.

Today your story begins again. Keep on sowing, being perseverant and you will overcome the obstacles in your path, cultivate your character, and create successes in your life.

Closing questions:

- What cultures and people do you identify with?

- Where are you on your hero's journey?

- What "boons" have you obtained and with whom can you share them?

- What emotional vices could you transcend into emotional virtues?

- Who would you be with a different story?

CHAPTER 2:

Finding Excellence: Habits, Practice, Philosophy and Love

"You are what you repeatedly do every day,
so whatever you're doing it's what you
become. If excellence is something you're
striving for, then it's not an accident,
it's a habit."
—Greg Plitt

- Habit: A behavior pattern acquired by frequent repetition or physiologic exposure that shows itself in regularity or increased facility of performance.
- Practice: To perform or work at repeatedly so as to become proficient; to train by repeated exercises.
- Philosophy: A particular set of ideas about knowledge, truth, the nature and meaning of life: a set of ideas about how to do something or how to live.

- Love: An intense feeling of deep affection.

ABOVE ARE THE definitions from the Webster Dictionary.[21] Simple and understandable. Here's my definitions and how I see the words.

- Habit: An action performed consciously or subconsciously frequently repeated causing increased or decreased performance toward achieving a particular outcome.

- Practice: Specific consistent action repeatedly performed to enhance abilities and develop skills thus creating habits.

- Philosophy: A person's belief based on knowledge from written texts, others experience, and personal experience of how to live.

- Love: A selfless giving of one's self and resources including time, energy, money, and knowledge accompanied by strong feelings of affection and gratitude for another person, activity, cause or yourself that is unconditional and resilient to outside forces of resistance.

I put two definitions for each word so as to give you contrast of the standard idea of what these words represent.

Seeing them from another standpoint may resonate with you. How we define our words and use the given meaning assigned to them will affect our outcomes. I encourage you to find the meaning of your words, particularly these four and see where they are benefiting you and where they are dragging you down. In the sections ahead we dive deep into what leading experts and philosophers have learned about habits and practice. We examine their philosophies based on experience and research and how love tethers them all together, supporting our habits, good and bad, and how they harmonize our bodies and minds resulting in Excellence.

Beginning with habits, the writer Samuel Johnson has captured the idea of how habits affect our life through a character named Theodore and a journey he takes up a mountain where habits are not intangible actions but rather little creatures that "ensnare our lives" on the road to the "Temple of Happiness".[22] I believe this story can afford an objective perspective to how we see our habits. Knowing this, it will make it easier to affect change in our actions beginning with awareness. Later in this tale of Habits we see how what we do will eventually determine where we end up, defining who we are. In his fictional examination, there are two possible outcomes. One ending in the "Caverns of Despair" ruled by a tyrant or the "Summit of Existence" where freedom reigns. His character Theodore, an old retired business man has returned to the mountainous countryside after a long career to reflect and live out his days until death takes him. One day, while taking care of his daily chores, he looks upon a rock overhanging where he lives that he hasn't climbed in years and has the desire to climb it again.

Once upon it, he felt compelled to go higher and higher, desiring to reach the summit as he had years before as a young man. Having not climbed in so long, feelings of fear and past experiences crept upon him along with a yearning for worthy work, for adventure, "the scenes of life" again. Having settled his anxious thoughts, he reflected about putting off this desire to climb for so long. He wonders if it has been laziness and not caution for not climbing this mountain he's been living under. Feeling ambitious again he decides to go on an adventure.

Rising early the next morning before the sun, he begins his ascent. Beginning ambitiously, he feels vitality coming back to him as he soaks in the nature around him. Soon though, he fatigues and decides to rest upon a small plain enclosed by rocks with beautiful views near the edge of a cliff where he can rest his head. In this place of peace, he falls asleep for what feels like a mere moment only to awaken to the sounds of eagles and a "being of more than human dignity" standing near him. This being asks what he's doing upon this cliff and after Theodore explains his why, the being says to look out over the ledge to see what isn't understood. "Look around, observe, contemplate and be instructed." Looking across the valley, Theodore sees another mountain. The Mountain of Existence. Looking closer into the valley at the base of the mountain are sweeping fields of flowers and grasses swaying in the breeze. To his surprise, men and women are down there hiking a path like his.

These people are with guides. The being standing with Theodore points them out as Innocence, Education, Reason, Religion, Pride and Conscious. Depending where they are on their ascent to the summit, they would team up with a particular guide. Those at the beginning of their journey would be with Innocence. She "seemed not overly solicitous to confine them to any settled pace or certain track; for she knew that the whole ground was smooth and solid, and that they could not easily be hurt or bewildered." This is like our beginnings. Mistakes are simply corrected and brushed by. They often mean very little when learning a new skill or performing a new task.

Next they travel with Education, "imperious in her commands, who confined them to certain paths, in their opinion too narrow and too rough." These are our parents, coaches and leaders guiding us from sending energy out in all directions and instead directing and channeling our energy into tasks that will make us proficient and skillful. Walking with Education is something that looked like pygmies or small beings, walking silently among them almost imperceptible to the human eye. They are smoothing the path for these new followers. These pygmies are called Habits.

As they walked with Education, she would frequently remind the group of these Habits and how they were ensnaring them with invisible chains and that they would have dominion over them. Some would grow in size to be bigger than them. Some habits would help and some would torture. Only as they neared the end of their journey would they know how the Habits would respond to them. With careful watch under Education, these Habits would follow quietly and would grow slowly, obeying commands and being all around helpful, steadily gaining mass and stature as they progressed on the journey. Being enticed by Appetites though, the hooligans of the valley, the Habits could grow to become massive quickly and lose their sense of service and humility and consequently abuse the follower.

Higher along the path, Education resigns her group to the next superior powers, next being Reason. A powerful guide with a demeanor that "appeared capable of presiding in senates, or governing nations". And Religion also known as Belief or Faith. Reason can only guide and cannot compel. It will not do more than it believes rational to do. Those who do not obey Reason will fall prey to Appetite and Passion, of which Lust and Vanity are the strongest. They would then be lured into the "Regions of Desire." Reason reminds the travelers about the path the followers choose: "The path seems now plain and even, but there are asperities and pitfalls, over which Religion [Faith] only can conduct you." Reason then passes those able over to Pride but only those not enslaved in the chains of bad Habits, under the rule of the tyrant of Despair can travel with her.

Even those on the straight and narrow are tempted sometimes. None are completely in the clear. Only those who stayed close to Reason and Faith, along with her emissary Conscience would climb higher. Those ensnared with bad Habits would be pulled back. Those who ignored Conscience, would without effect, fail to break their chains of bad habits. "Even with Faith nearby, they could not join her, though they wanted to walk with her and hated their habits". With every attempt, the Habits would pull them back and lash them.

The Good Habits, now larger and stronger, would work together with the guides to pull the follower up steep slopes of adversity and chaotic conditions they encountered on the climb. Those who learned, then implemented the teachings of Reason and Faith were set free one chain at a time and directed to the Temple of Happiness on the summit. Seeing this all unfold, the guide Theodore stands with encourages him to withdraw from the cliff he's standing, the "Regions of Obscurity" and see the fates of those who didn't listen. He says "Take heed and be instructed."

Taking a short walk to get another view, he looked into the other land nearby. These were the Caverns of Despair and Misery, Desire and Sadness and watched the people there for a moment carrying on without pleasure in their progress and without a way to return to the Road of Reason and reach the summit. Their final place was in the hands of Melancholy and once she was done torturing her prisoner, she would turn them over to the cruel tyrant of Despair to finish them off. The guide then yells, startling Theodore: "Be wise and let not Habit prevail against thee." To which Theodore awakens and realizes it's a dream. He has insights now.

The moral of the story is this:

Just as this once young business man grew into old age, we too are growing older with one less day in our future and one more day in our past. If we keep doing the old things that don't work, we will keep getting the same results, beginning a descent into the Caverns of Despair or like Theodore, we can start climbing our mountain. By making the choice to climb, everyday is a day we grow higher and stronger just like the Good Habits that surround the travelers. This will be hard. We will have to change some things in our life. Some things and people will no longer fit in our life, our routines. We will have to **exercise discipline daily.** We will encounter fear and passions and problems all along the way but by being committed to growing, to learning and educating ourselves, we will find a way through these obstacles to our Summit of Happiness. We don't have to serve our Habits, our habits can serve us. It's worthy work.

Breaking the Bad: Building the Good

Our routines, as mundane as they seem constitute a majority of our life. Researchers estimate that habits make up to 40 to 50 percent of our actions on any given day. Because of this we are limited by our habits and where they lead us. Each day is made up of many moments but stem from only a few habit patterns. Each pattern setting the path of how our next moment, day, week and year will go. The little ignorances we perform by accident or even out of bad practice could one day be fatal to you or others. Knowing how much habits control our daily lives, how do we break away from the bad habits slowing us down from progressing and begin forming new efficient habits? The first answer is our psychology.

What we think affects what we do. Our results reflect our actions. James Clear illustrates in his compelling book, Atomic Habits using what he Calls the Four Laws to both break and build good habits.[23]

1) Cue
2) Craving
3) Response
4) Reward

<u>Cues</u>

A cue is a signal that triggers a behavior or thought to initiate an action. Every cue is a signal to a potential reward.
Time, environment, event, emotions, and people are cues
that have rewards linked to them. Have you ever tried to
sleep in past your usual wake up time for work? You lay
in bed on the weekend for the next hour trying to get the
extra sleep only to be held awake by your body clock, yet
you keep trying because you know extra sleep feels good
or maybe you reach for snack at 11 am even when your
not hungry but only because you read the clock and the
thought of food creates a craving. The environment we
live and work in dictates responses from us too. Home is
usually a place of calm and quiet where we can in essence
"breathe" after a long day. That's rewarding. At the gym,
being around motivated, fired up individuals inspires you.
You may be tired but you do one more set. You feel pulled
to do more. Though both places are different, the reward
is the same. A change in state. One to come down and one
to come up.

For anyone who has felt moments of compassion for
a friend or deep loss of a relationship knows emotions are
powerful. You feel them even when it's not happening to
you like when watching a film or seeing people reunite at
the airport. When we personally experience feelings either
directly or empathetically regularly, we begin to wire ourselves for more of that experience. The saying "birds of a

feather flock together" applies here. Negatives are easy to fall into because they take less effort and are immediately rewarding, they change our state quickly, though they crush the individual's potential on the backend. Positive emotions can become a norm but that will take some work. We have to earn it.

Events like test taking or our phone buzzing are cues for us to take action and find rewards. The teacher passes out the final test and you've studied. You know the material inside and out. You want the "A", the gold star. It raises our status in the class, inside ourselves and opens avenues of opportunity. That's rewarding. "Dinggggg" says the IPhone. We want to open the message. We want to "connect". It feels good having people reach out.

People's presence are some of the most powerful cues. You're in the gym and Miss yoga pants walks by, she smiles and waves. You smile back and may even approach to chat, catch up, connect. Friendships are being formed or maybe you've been dropping the weights in the back of the gym during yoga class on Mondays. The nice lady upfront that warned you three times not to do that is now on a warpath. She's coming at you. Fast. You may now have the craving or desire to clean up and evacuate the building before she tears you a new page.

Cues are meaningless until interpreted by a person in the context of their past experience. The same event or person may evoke a totally different response based on what has been their result before.

Cravings

Cravings are the motivational force behind every habit. Remove this step and there's no reason to act. We may see the reward but if it doesn't stimulate the need for the feeling we desire (pleasure) or the need to avoid pain we won't do anything about it. **Every craving is linked to a desire to change an internal state.** Cravings, like cues, are contextual. They vary greatly from person to person because the information or experience they have is subjective. The sound of clanking weights at the gym for some people fires them up to get in the rack, for others that may be obnoxious. An old country song comes on the radio, someone is motivated to do some dosie dough, another wants to drive his truck into a wall because it reminds him of his ex-girlfriend. Same song, different craving of state change.

Response

Response is the actual routine performed. This can be in the form of thought too. The phone dings and your first thought is it's your spouse. She has been flirting all day. She's on your mind. It can also be a physical action. Your training partner throws a right hook, you bob and counter with a left hook and right cross. A response requires two things:

- Ability
- Effort

If either are lacking the response won't happen. For example, if you want to surf but you don't have the balance to stand on the board, you won't build the habit of carving in the waves. If it is too hard to get the board out of the garage because it's cluttered, the ocean is an hour away, and you drive a car that won't fit the board on top, the amount of effort to surf is likely to outweigh the reward even if you know how to surf or want to surf.

Reward

You finish your workout. Today was a high intensity, reps for days type workout. One thing is on your mind, food. What kind? Simple carbs, something sweet. Why? There's energy there. Dopamine will be released. You now head home to rendezvous with post workout ambrosia. You see the house, slight anticipation builds. More dopamine. Once inside you get all the ingredients out. You get it all in the blender and realize no water bottles, no almond milk. F. Cortisol rises and dopamine falls. You begin the hunt around the house. You check the stash spot and volía, there's one there. Back in the game baby. You mix it up and then swig it back. Satisfaction washes over you. Reward centers are lighting up. Reward chemicals are flowing. Your brain just learned where (the house) and how (the shake) to refuel again. The actions taken are being reinforced.

Where do rewards begin? They begin in the brain. The hot spots for rewards and feel good chemicals are the <u>ventral</u>

tegmental area (VTA), where dopamine is produced. The dorsal striatum is a cluster of neurons that form habits by identifying pleasurable patterns like where to get your post workout meal or hot sex with your partner. The prefrontal cortex plays a role by interacting with dopamine and creating visual images of the reward. Just to clarify though, more than, dopamine is involved in the pathways of reward and pleasure. Dopamine is just a major contributor and for the context of this book and for simplicity it is mentioned in this section.

Rewards do two things: (1) they serve to satisfy our craving and (2) teach us where to continue to get these items. Rewards are both tangible and intangible. There are things like food, money, and sex. The secondary rewards of these things are access to resources, fame, status, praise and approval from others, love and friendship, and feelings of personal confidence.

Not all rewards are created equal though. Eating a doughnut now may taste good and be satisfying for a moment. The guilt it brings on later by the added weight, belly ache and brain fog will not be so rewarding. The guy or gal who's available tonight while your partner is away but will be gone tomorrow, will leave you worse mentally, emotionally and reputationally than if you held the line on your discipline. Why then do we repeat things that harm us?

The ratio of pain to pleasure it brought on was not great enough to tip the balance. The pain fades quickly but you still remember the reward. When the reward is great enough, the feedback will continue the cycle encouraging us to repeat the process. The reward circuits are still there. Literal neurons are laid down. New circuits have to be built or rewired or the old ones destroyed. Cues don't even have to register consciously to cause us to act. A study by Anna Rose Childress found that people who are addicted to drugs don't have to consciously register a cue for it to arouse their reward system. In a study published in PLoS One, she scanned the brains of twenty-two recovering cocaine addicts while photos of crack pipes and other drug paraphernalia flashed before their eyes for *thirty-three milliseconds*, one-tenth the time it takes to blink. The men didn't consciously see anything, but the images activated the same parts of the reward neurons that visible drug cues excite.

An old method used in a new way is being performed by Dr. Gallimberti and colleagues using what is known as Transcranial magnetic stimulation (TMS). This alters electrical activity in brain areas that cause craving and desire, thus acticativing other neural pathways that reverse addiction. They tested in 2016 with twenty-nine people. Sixteen in the TMS group and thirteen in the control group with standard care. By the end of the trials, eleven of the sixteen were drug-free while only three in the control group of thirteen became drug-free.

So whether you're trying to break a bad food habit, kick the obsessive phone checking habit or even stop using legal and illegal substances, remove the cues that used to be rewarding. Though you cannot "see" them, your brain can.

Your body can. **Make taking the proper action easy.** If the things you are doing are not working, seek the professionals that can help you. The rewards it brings will reward you and your loved ones fruitfully.

So next time instead of grabbing for a donut, you opt for an apple or sweet potato, know that dopamine and serotonin still get released, just not as quickly. Your body responds rather than reacts to the sugar because of the fiber. Now you stay lean and your ability to think remains clear. It's thinking in sequential order. The first order consequence usually sucks but the second, third and beyond consequences are much more rewarding. For example, going to the gym and working out will make you sore. Not ideal. Second order consequence of that is healing and getting stronger. The third order consequence is changing your body aesthetically. Then you start thinking clearer. People start treating you differently. Then you start acting differently. Your life begins to change for the better.

And when you fall short of your mark, and we will— life challenges our routine— Murphy will come knocking on your door or head soon and that's natural. The difference between winning and losing though is showing up, being consistent, particularly the days you don't "feel" like it or you're tired or sore. You miss a workout because of a celebration, it happens. Work late once and miss family time, it happens. Miss two workouts, work late again and you are sowing the seeds of failure. A new habit is being created.

And if you encounter anything troublesome or pleasant or glorious or inglorious, remember that the hour of struggle has come, the Olympic contest is here and you may put off no longer, and that one day and one action determines whether the progress you have achieved is lost or maintained.

-Epictetus

<u>Failure:</u> A few errors in judgment repeated everyday.

<u>Success:</u> A few simple disciplines practiced everyday.

For me, workouts and diet are most valuable to who I am and who I am becoming. Integrating that in my early years was simple because of the frustrations and the environment I was in. Reading has become the same way. Even if I'm tired, sore, haven't slept or eaten, I show up and go through the motions just to keep the feeling of progress. The actions, the workout, the meal, the reading is a reward in itself. When acting on the things you know are good for you becomes rewarding in and of itself, you will have more satisfaction in your life.

Observe what habits you have now, seek out and imagine what habits you want to build and which ones you wish to break by following these principles. The key is awareness. If you can identify it, you have the potential to change it. You get to change it. It's yours. Own it. You have material to work with. Make the routine or behavior easy to do, keep them in front of you and elicit people in your circle to hold you accountable. When you fall off track, they will give the nudges you need to walk your path to the best you.

Habit A&P

The answers to how we form habits are in our anatomy and physiology. Our Brain contains three major sections earning the name: The Triune Brain.

- Neocortex
- Limbic Brain
- Reptilian brain (cerebellum)

The neocortex or thinking brain, is the seat of our conscious awareness. It's the newest addition to our anatomy and is used for gathering information and reining in our emotions. It's the charioteer in Phaedrus and Reason in the Story of Habit. It's divided into four lobes. Frontal, Parietal, Temporal, and Occipital. Covering the brain like a rind on a fruit. Every time we learn something new, we make new synaptic connections in the neocortex. In reading a new book, learning a new technique in the gym, learning a new language, confronting a fear or learning a new emotion and repeating this behavior, our brain is literally upgrading its hardware to support its software. Hardware being the neurons themselves and software being the knowledge and meaning assigned to it. The more we repeat an action or activity, the more readily the neurons fire together, strengthening their connection. This was discovered by Donald Hebb in 1949 and is referred to as Hebb's Law.

In short, **Neurons that fire together wire together.**

The limbic brain is a complex set of structures found on the central underside of the cerebrum. It is responsible for the integration of our emotional lives with our higher mental functions, such as learning or retaining information in the short term and long term as memories. It's why eating is pleasurable and why we feel fear and love. This system propagates those feelings. This system contains the amygdala, hippocampus, thalamus, hypothalamus, basal ganglia, and cingulate gyrus.

The reptilian brain or the cerebellum is the seat of our subconscious brain. It's the oldest part of the brain, meaning it was with us before we became Homo sapiens. It controls our vital functions like breathing, heart rate and where impulsive and compulsive behaviors stem from. It regulates motor movements, balance, posture, coordination and speech. Only making up 10% of an average brain weight, it accounts for more than 50% of all the neurons in the brain.

All together the brain is made up of approximately 100 billion neurons with over 100 trillion synaptic connections that are both local and span long distances. Neurons communicate electrically and chemically. Electricity is used by the brain to control ion flows which allow the cells to process and store information. That information is then literally wired into our biological architecture. **Learning is building new synaptic connections and remembering is strengthening those synaptic connections.**

1,000 days of practice
10,000 days of refinement

-Miyamoto Musashi

The more the neurons fire together and wire together they begin to create networks of synaptic connections known as neural networks. It's like an IT room. The building being the brain and the IT room is the network of neurons. Each level of the building has an IT room and the cable in them represents an individual neuron or nerve cell. The amount of activity in the rooms surrounding the IT room of the building determines the amount of cables for that room. The more activity, the more cables. In rooms unused, cables get demoed out, "pruned" away or rerouted to support other areas just like in our brain.

Scientifically speaking, the mind is what our brain does. For us, that means our habits are our mind and our mind is our brain and we can take conscious control of some of that. We can make the brain fire in different sequences from the ones we are currently experiencing. **Our habits**

are therefore networks of densely myelinated neurons and when we recall or perform a habit, we fire those neurons making them stronger. By modifying our behavior, changing our actions, we have a new experience. This experience is now a foundation for new neural connections. In this new experience of the five senses, our brain begins forming neural connections for the new experience by releasing chemicals in the limbic brain we know as feelings and emotions.

This is how we remember our first kiss, the birth of our child, graduation or even the death of a loved one. Now this describes novel moments. Routine on the other hand, after a while communicates to the brain that it's okay not to consciously remember vivid details of an experience. It becomes subconscious and the reason for that is once routine becomes habit, it frees the brain to focus on other tasks, to learn new skills.

For many years, scientists believed that these neural connections were fixed when we reached adulthood. If cells of the brain died, that was it. In recent years, science has demonstrated that our brains can grow new neurons and though as adults, our brains are not nearly as plastic as a child or adolescent, our brains still retain plasticity or the ability to shape to changing circumstances and environments. It's how people like James Clear recovered from his massive brain injury and it's how I recovered from my minor concussions. To be clear, this doesn't mean the affected brain will be normal again. Just because we can regenerate, doesn't mean we will be near what we were before we experienced a tragedy or injury. Keeping with brain plasticity, we can adapt to the changing circumstances taking what Dave Brailsford, the Olympic British cycling coach calls 1% improvements.

The One Percenters

> "The whole principle came from the idea that if you broke down everything you could think of that goes into riding a bike, and then improve it by 1%, you'll get a significant increase when you put them all together."
> —Dave Brailsford

This philosophy is known as the Aggregation of marginal gains: The search for a marginal improvement in everything you do.

In 2003, David Brailsford was hired as the new performance director in charge of coaching the Professional British Cycling Team called Team Sky. In the last century up until 2003, the British cycling team had only won one gold medal. One, at the Olympic Games and had no wins ever in the Tour de France. The reason Brailsford was hired was his unique philosophy. He's microfocused.

He looked for one percent improvements everywhere. From massage gels for faster muscle recovery, the best pillows to sleep with, the best way to wash their hands to prevent colds and infections are just a few examples. Over a period of five years, these small changes made an exponential impact on the results of their races. In the 2008 Beijing games they won 14 medals, 8 of which were gold, claiming 60 percent of all medals won that year. In the same year, Bradley Wiggins was the first to win the Tour de France for the British cycling team. The team then won the next year. In the years following, the team won the 2015, 2016, and 2017 races, earning five victories in six years. You may not want to ride your bike as much as these guys do but we all could benefit from increased performance in our lives.

By increasingly getting better at an activity by one percent every day, in one year we will end up thirty-seven times better. Do the math. Remember, the small things are the big monumental things. If bad habits announce themselves to you, or when you become aware of them, see if you can correct what you are doing. We must begin fixing the things we repeat everyday. **The things we repeat daily are the most important things, however small.** They create who we are in our eyes and others. It determines the direction of our life. There's a rule in flying airplanes called 1 in 60. For every one degree your off target, you will end up sixty miles off your destination. If you were to start at the equator and fly the equator belt around the world, one degree off would put you 400 miles off your initial destination. That gap difference is the distance between Baltimore and South Carolina.

So where do you start? Where you are right now.

Consider the *two-minute rule* by David Allen. This rule states that when starting a new habit, it should take no longer than two minutes to do. Here are some examples. You want to read two books a month. This now becomes reading before bed for 10 minutes. You want to go to the gym more after work then becomes, get your gym clothes on when you get home. Think of two things you could change in your immediate environment or just today in general. One mental way to make approaching the process easier is by saying you "get to" rather than "have to" do something.

Then let's say you fix your bedtime, then your breakfast, making bed time one hour earlier by turning out the lights and leaving your phone in another room once it's dark out. You put healthy food out before bed like oatmeal so it's easier to make in the morning. I guarantee if you do this for one week, your life will begin to transform. Then keep doing it. Keep molding your habits to make them the way you need them to be to win the next moment, the next hour, the next day. These changes are marginal, almost indiscernible but like a plane one degree off course, one habit can change your desired destination.

Another perspective is water turning into steam. At 99°C there is no change. It's water. Hot, scolding but no transformation. One more degree and it's in a totally new form. How do we get there? One degree at a time. Lao Tzu once said, the journey of one thousand miles begins with one step. You cannot leap there or even fly there without doing mile one then two then three and so on. It's a daily process. This takes persistence and patience. One day away or a thousand miles away, with one step, one rep, you are closer.

For you hunters out there, there's one more way to relay this message. While training for the military and as a kid growing up, I shot a lot of weapons. One thing I was taught in the programs and by experienced rifle men was the natural point of aim. The Natural point of aim is when you and your rifle are together at rest. You do this by taking a deep breath and focusing on your front sight. Then you release this breath. At the end of the breath, focused on the front sight, you and your weapon are at your natural point of aim. When you squeeze the trigger, the bullet will land on that point. Habit change is like the resetting of your natural point of aim. We go the direction we focus on, the direction of our habits. To become someone new, to do more than what we are doing now, we have to reset our habits.

Habits are Long Done

The Chinese bamboo tree takes 5 years to break the surface of the earth and requires watering and nurturing daily. Once sprouted, in five weeks it grows ninety feet tall. A zen story illustrates this well:

One morning a zen disciple comes to the garden of the monastery. Ch'anyom, an older disciple, plants a patch of bamboo trees and begins to water them. He tells the new disciple Dario, about the bamboo tree and it's magnificent growth and strength. Hearing of this, he runs to the neighboring village and gets one the same morning and plants it on the other side of the garden. Weeks pass. Months pass. Seasons change. With regularity and consistency, Ch'anyom waters and speaks kind words to these bamboo trees. Dario does the same. Then suddenly Dario, watering his tree, throws his water pale down and walks over to Ch'anyom and belittles his actions. "What nonsense are we doing? Watering this patch of earth? And of what are our results? For months we have been watering and not even weeds have sprouted here."

Ch'anyom with wise eyes, smiles, finishes watering the patch of earth and with a low voice says "every day, in every way, we are closer and closer. Though we cannot see the result, the happening is happening. Persistence is the key."

Dario scoffs with bravado and leaves the garden. Every day, Ch'anyom shows up watering the plant, nurturing, loving, tending. Dario from across the garden shows up still but now just to watch, spout doubts and deter the actions of the other.

5 years pass. Small sprouts appear. Ch'anyom with warmth in his voice welcomes this new life. Dario, passing by, just laughs hysterically.

"5 years and this? These are your trees? Your labor of love was wasted." And walks away, leaving to meditate in a neighboring village.

5 weeks pass.

Dario returns to the temple and finds it empty. He begins looking for the other disciples but cannot find any of them anywhere. He hears sounds of playful banter and cheerful conversation coming from the garden and sees massive Bamboo stalks coming from outside the garden walls. He runs over, wide eyed and bewildered.

"Ch'anyom, who's trees are these? Who put them there?

"They are the same ones planted 5 years ago. I have planted them here." Ch'anyom said. "The same time you planted yours."

Dario looks to the place he planted.

Ch'anyom says, "It seems that, like your tree, you have not grown. If we are to make progress, we must water daily, nurture daily. Plant again. Be consistent and be aware of the changes occurring beyond our eyes. Five years will pass quickly, plant again. The time will pass anyway. Plant again. Just be consistent and aware.

Final Words on Habits

At the end of our habits are results. Results matter. To get the results you want, you have to form the habits. We are not always after the end result though. That's a one time victory. Life isn't just one game you win and call yourself victorious. It's a series of games we must win over and over and over ad infinitum if we are to achieve excellence and fulfillment in our lives. The habits we form through repetition that continue to return desired results without conscious thought is the true result we are after. What Dr. Joe Dispenza calls going from thinking to doing, to being.

So **even when you don't feel like it, do the thing you have to do.** In fact, that's when you most need to do it. It's your old way of taking action trying to keep a neuronal path open. Keep going. You may think "this one time won't matter much" and you're probably right. One more time in that moment likely won't change much. But just because nothing has happened yet doesn't mean it's not happening. It's still at a quantum level. There's a lag in our awareness of the energy and processes at work in our body. It hasn't reached the threshold of our awareness yet. It's working though. **Your actions matter.** Some more than others but they all carry weight. Things will improve, even if it's one percent. That's forward progress. Stay the course.

On Practice

> The only conclusive evidence of a man's sincerity is that he gives himself for a principle. Words, money, all things else are comparatively easy to give away; but when a man makes a gift of his daily life and practice, it is plain that the truth,

whatever it may be, has taken possession of him.
—Lowell

The Success Library

<u>We Gotta Keep It Myelinated</u>

How do professionals maintain a high level of performance? They train daily. Many people train daily though and don't create the same effect, the same result. What is it that makes them great? How is excellence maintained? The answer is in our Myelin.

Myelin is a mixture of proteins and phospholipids forming a whitish insulating sheath around many nerve fibers, increasing the speed at which impulses are conducted. It works like the cabling in our electronics, keeping the electrical signal strong by preventing it from leaking out. Not as sexy as it looks on the field but it's where the real magic happens. When we practice playing an instrument, kicking a ball, training a movement in the gym we are actually wrapping our neurons, specifically our axons with myelin. With every wrap we increase our skill and the speed at which we perform. The thicker the sheath, the faster electrical impulses can travel, the more accurate we become in our movement and thinking.

So how is this fatty substance myelin made? It's made by a combination of cells in the brain known as *astrocytes, oligodendrocytes, and schwann cells.* If you've ever held a brain or dissected one in biology class you know that it's firm but not hard. Partially because it's been embalmed but also because of astrocytes. Astrocytes give structure to the brain while also releasing chemicals that produce, maintain and develop both our neurons and glia. They constitute between 25% to 50% of cellular volume in a majority of brain areas.

Neuron Anatomy

Being how voluminous astrocytes are in the brain, they act to maintain the extracellular milieu that surrounds neurons during their firing or transmission. They promote the uptake of excitatory neurotransmitters like dopamine, norepinephrine (brain adrenaline) and epinephrine (adrenaline). In short, astrocytes support the structure and firing of the neurons and help absorb the chemicals released by the cells.

The two cells that actually produce the sheaths you see above are the **oligodendrocytes** and **schwann cells**, also known as **supporter cells**. These cells sense when the nerves fire and respond to the firing neuron by wrapping myelin on the nerves that fires. The more a nerve fires, the more myelin wraps it. The more wraps it gets, the faster the nerve transmission is, sometimes firing 200 mph or faster.

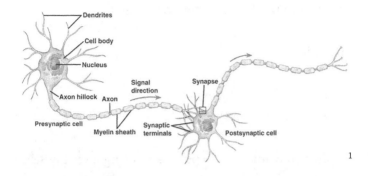

"As a single footstep will not make a path on
the earth, so a single thought will not make a
pathway in the mind. To make a deep physical
path, we walk again and again on that ground.
To make a deep mental path, we must think over
and over again the kinds of thoughts we wish to
dominate our lives.
—Unknown

Those players we see on the gridiron, in the cage, in the
olympic arena have developed, through years of consistent
proper practice, many layers of myelin. Some have genetic
advantages of height or weight, sure but overall what separates an average performance from extraordinary is how
insulated the habit-pattern circuit is. This is how Kobe
Bryant hits so many shots, how Tom Brady makes so many
good throws to his teammates, how Roy Jones Jr. could out
maneuver and strike down opponents in the ring.

---

[1] https://askabiologist.asu.edu/neuron-anatomy

So how can we develop extraordinary skills?

Two things:

1) Inspiration
2) Deep Practice

Inspiration defined is the process of being mentally stimulated to do or feel something, particularly something creative. It's your fuel.

Deep practice is defined as stopping when errors occur, practicing that one skill until it's mastered then continuing the process until it's finished or completed. This is the actual work of building wraps of myelin. This will take a long time but is less time than not doing it at all.

The Fire Within

I had a soccer coach growing up that was from England. Before every game he would huddle us up and set the tone before the match. One of the things he said before he set us out on the field was "play with passion." As American kids we just loved the accent but reflecting back to what he said and how he said it, it fired us up too. Even when we lost, when we gave it our all, we felt accomplished because we left everything on the field. We were growing our potential for the next game.

So what has you fired up to grow? Where do you want to get better or what has you pulled in a direction that no one can deter you from? It likely has had a major effect on the direction of your life and will come quickly to mind. It's tied to your identity. It's tied to deep emotions and images of your ideal self and reality. It's the thing your inner voice says to you "that's who I want to be."

That thing is your inspiration. Cultivate that. You will need it. You will need it because it's going to take years to develop into a professional, approximately ten years of dedicated practice. What Ander Ericsson calls the 10,000 hour rule.[37] In that time there will be setbacks and days where things don't go right. Circumstances suck or people don't come through and what will keep you going is your love of the thing itself, the inner fire of inspiration.

> "Our inward power, when it obeys nature, reacts
> to events by accommodating itself to what it faces
> - to what is possible. It needs no specific material.
> It pursues its own aims as circumstances allow;
> it turns obstacles into fuel. As a fire overwhelms
> what would have quenched a lamp, what's thrown
> on top of the conflagration is absorbed, consumed
> by it - and makes it burn still higher."
> —Marcus Aurelius

The Primal Signals

People often think their inspiration started with them but in fact it came from cues that triggered a response in our biology. As children, before words had a major significance, we thought in terms of images.

Inspiration could have come from a film, from a teacher, from a concert, or witnessing an act of kindness or even malevolence. The key is that it inspired action, a want to change your inner state and outward circumstances and create an environment and reality beyond where you stand now.

More often than is known, most successful people in history had major tragic events happen to them at an early age or grew up in rough neighborhoods or environments while their brains were still developing. People like Curtis Jackson (50 cent) who lost his mom at age 8 and grew up in drug infested and gang saturated Queens, Julius Caesar losing his father at 15 and being captured by pirates at age 25, Nietzsche losing his father at age 4, Epictetus being born into slavery, beaten and crippled and going on to have a successful career in politics. This gave them a strong reason and desire to work harder and commit more to getting out of where they were, emotionally and physically and into a better environment. This isn't always the case though. "The same water that hardens the egg, softens the carrot."

Depending on how this individual frames the situation as they grow older and the people they surround themselves with, will determine whether they take the high road of commited practice, of their passion or the low road of the appetites to drown their pains. Now if you haven't had a major life crisis event happen, don't make one. View history and let empathy affect you. Just by hearing the stories and circumstances that others come from can be enough to ignite the fire of inspiration inside you to act.

Mad Skills

All the people who develop the most skills over time possess three qualities:

- Energy
- Passion
- Commitment

Energy to practice and maintain the drive to practice consistently. Passion that makes them fanatic about the art or practice and becoming this new identity and commitment to stay the course when progress is slow and your body hurts or mind is tired.

Deep Practice | Unhurried Intensity

Better to believe yourself a dunce and work hard,
than a genius and work idle.
—The Success Library

When doing anything you can practice deep practice. To keep it simple, let's say you're playing a guitar. The song is the National Anthem. Simple. Playing the first section is smooth. Coming into the second section, you play the first note sharp. Pause. Look at the music. Play that one note in isolation. Feeling how you pluck the string, how your fingers slide to the next chord. You back up and play the section before. You miss it again. You again pluck the cord. Find the proper placement and play it together. You nail it. You go back and nail it again. Then you play this way all the way through.

That's deep practice.

This can be done with workouts, with vocabulary, with music, with any skill you want to develop. The essential elements of deep practice are:

1) Segmenting
   a) Learn from a Master
   b) Macro to Micro: Absorb Everything
   c) Slow and Steady

2) Repetition
   a) Quality Practice: Time
   b) Consistent Practice
   c) Feedback from a Master

3) Concentrate
    a) Feel the Mistake
    b) Feel the Way

4) Sleep
    a) Stages of sleep and how it affects our performance
    b) Sleep spindles and learning

Put another way, deep practice is an unhurried intensity. You're moving slowly but with intense focus, deliberate action. It's consistent quality movement and thinking in a deliberate way done quantitatively that brings about a particular result that you know will be produced. It's like learning to maneuver in your room in the dark. You know what's there and in a sense where things are but in the dark it's like a new environment. You bump the edge of the bed. You stop, think and move forward a little more. Occasionally you step on something, maybe you trip but once you have done this one hundred, two hundred...three thousand times, you get an intuitive feel almost as if the light has come on and you work effortlessly through what were once obstacles. You have created a mental map.

Learn from a Master

When you want to improve, what do you do first? Find a model that's winning, that's successful in your eyes and emulate their style. You copy until you can create. You follow in their footsteps until you find your own style. Inspiration begins here then morphs into obsessive practice, deep practice, deliberate practice. The grand vision of your best self begins to form and you now have the first part of practice, the Macro.

Macro

The first step to deep practice is seeing the macro, the whole task, the whole movement, then segmenting it so you can digest each piece. For example a clean and press.

Micro

The second step is dividing the whole up into smaller parts called micros. Micros are the movements or ideas that make up the entire task. As for a clean and press that would be the initial deadlift to high pull. From high pull to moving under the bar to front squat. From front squat to standing. Standing to press.

Slow and Steady

The third step is executing the movement slowly until you feel the nuances of the movement and can control the weight then you do it in real time all together.

This is how people like Nick Saban, coach of Alabama football, breaks down film. He spends hours and hours during the week watching other teams best plays off the line, in a throw, at the goal line. Then he watches his own team's strategic play's in the same way. Studying the movements and patterns of the teams coming up and of his current players skills in a micro way then piecing it together allows him to hone the patterns to beat his opponents by landslides.

For events like music that often are less filmed and more often audio recorded, it's listening and feeling the music. When possible, watching the player pluck strings or beat the drums or draw the bow of a violin. Next is visualizing yourself performing in your mind's eye then actually playing the selected piece of music section by section, correcting errors along the way until it's flawless. Glenn Kurtz in his book *Practicing* describes the feeling of practicing while playing music: "Each day, with every note, practicing is the same task, this essential human gesture--reaching out for an idea, for the grandeur of what you desire, and feeling it slip through your fingers." That last part keeps pulling you back in to master the next step, to continue to hit the sweet spot of your craft, to continue to consistently practice.

In deep practice, form and technique are the main emphasis. If you can do it well slowly, you will do it exceptionally fast later. In MMA training my coach would always remind us, "slow is smooth, smooth is fast." The reason we go slow is that it takes time for the body to register that it needs to wrap myelin for that pattern, that circuit. This could take days and weeks to begin and years to thicken and become prominent in the brain. The next key is consistency. The same is true in the other direction. It only requires a skilled person to stop firing his or her circuits for thirty days for the myelin to stop wrapping and deteriorate from that circuit. Daily practice matters, particularly as we get older. Being that our myelin is a living tissue, it's always being broken down and repaired. As we age this process gets slower, with deterioration becoming more prominent. Gaps then form within our neural insulation. This is why older people move more slowly. The muscles haven't changed much but the myelin is thinner or has gaps. This makes their signals slower.

"If I don't practice one day, I know it; two days, the critics know it; three days, the public knows it."
—Jascha Heifetz

Another saying you may have heard is "muscle memory". It's not that our muscles remember what we did. They don't. We consciously do in our mind but it's the speed at which our impulses fire into those neural networks in the muscles that brings the results back quickly because they already have a certain number of layers of myelin laid down and since they fire faster than the other circuits they get more myelin again faster than a new circuit. On the reverse side of aging, you may hear old people out performing young people and they should. They had more time, more sleep and more training to grow and lay down myelin. If they have taken proper care of themselves, they have every reason to perform excellently.

Repetition: Quality

Quality repetitions are the key. Doing a set of squats with poor form will either cause injury or improper development. No circuit will be built for high performance. Bouncing around from page to page reading and not focusing on the main objective of the book won't lead to more understanding. It's too novel. The key is **quality repetitions across consistent sets of time.**

What this means is your form or technique has to be proper. Then keeping that rhythm until performance starts to wane, beyond that point practice won't make you better but potentially worse because you aren't practicing the proper thing anymore. Anders Ericsson, a professional in the study of human performance says "To maximize gains from long-term practice, individuals must avoid exhaustion and must limit practice to an amount from which they can completely recover on a daily or weekly basis."

On average the block of time for an adult in one session of deep practice is about one hour, performed 3 to five days a week. For children the time is lower, approximately ten to twenty minutes a day, three to five days a week until they adapt and improve. Practice can then be extended. Studies have shown no benefit from durations exceeding four hours per day and reduced benefits from practice exceeding two hours at a time. C. E. Seashore, a researcher in music psychology, once stated, "Many a student becomes disgusted with music because he cannot learn by dull drudgery. **The command to rest is fully as important as to work in effective learning.**" C.E Seashore goes on to say that practice should be less than one hour with ample rest in between practice. Another great musician named Leopold Auer was once asked "How long should one practice?"

To which professor Auer replied:

"The right kind of practice is not a matter of hours. Practice should represent the utmost concentration of the brain. It is better to play with concentration for two hours than to practice eight without. I should say that four hours would be a good maximum practice."

In the observation of Olympic swimmers, Daniel Chambliss, Yale graduate and author of *The Making of an Olympic Swimmer* noted "the secret to attaining excellence is always to maintain close attention to every detail of performance, each one done correctly, time and time again, until excellence in every detail becomes a firmly ingrained habit."

Consistency

In a study of violinists at the Music Academy of West Berlin, three groups of ten people were created. One considered the best violinists, considered to become international soloists, the second, the good violinists, and the third were called music teachers because they were unlikely to become international soloists.

Each violinist was interviewed during three sessions of interviews. During the first session they were asked about the start of practice, sequence of music teachers, and participation in competitions. The students were then asked to estimate how many hours per week they had practiced alone with the violin for each year since they had started to practice.

During the second session, the violinists answered questions about practice and concentration. Every violinist was asked to keep a diary and journal the activities they performed over the course of a 24-hour day in 15-minute intervals and asked to rate 0-10 the relevance of the activity to their performance and then rate the effort required to perform the activity. They did this for 7-full days. The third interview was discussing activity related to performance.

What was discovered was, on average the best violinist began playing around age 8, and decided to become musicians around age 15. Each of the best violinists had an average of 4 music teachers or mentors and studied 2 other instruments. 27 out of 30 violinists gave practice the highest relevant rating compared to playing for fun which received a lower rating. Of the controllable music related activities for the day: practice was the most relevant. The best violinist rated the practice alone the highest and practiced an average of 3.5 hours a day, everyday. The music teachers only practice 1.3 hours a day. The best and good violinists practiced alone before lunch between the hours of 10 am and 2 pm whereas the music teachers had no pattern of practice.

There are a couple take-aways here. One, keep a journal. Know what activities you are doing and why. Ask yourself: "Is what I am about to do or am currently doing going to maximize my performance later?" We can only manage what we can measure. In building 11, the Power Plant of the National Institute of Health, there is a quote in big bold letters on the back wall of the command center posted, " **You can't manage what you can't measure.**" We can only take control of what we are aware of. Seeing it written keeps us aware and begins to make it real. The second takeaway is the best; **stay consistent.** They make practice a daily part of their routines. Now, you may not want to practice violin but you have to practice that which you desire to excel in. If not to become professional, just for the sake of your brain health. Studies show that by engaging your brain in challenging ways, say playing crossword puzzles, reduces onset of Alzheimer's by 2.54 years compared to those who didn't play or practice crossword puzzles. Engage your brain. Step up to a challenge again and again. You will thank yourself later. So will that boy, that girl and the people you care about. People you don't know yet are rooting for you and counting on your successes.

Hey DJ Feed that Back

One of the most critical things in learning and getting better is feedback. In the absence of adequate feedback, efficient learning is not possible and improvements are minimal even for highly motivated individuals. Just doing repetitions of an activity will not automatically lead to improvement or accuracy of performance. The best way to do your reps is with someone who's experienced and who knows the way in a one-on-one atmosphere. Studies have shown that **individualized supervision by a teacher is superior.** When students were assigned either a conventional teaching method in a group setting or a tutor teaching with a conventional method, the average tutoring student performed in the 98th percentile.

One thing more about practice and repetition, engaging in deliberate practice generates no immediate monetary rewards and will actually generate costs associated with access to teachers, coaches, mentors and training environments. For example, International-level performers often receive their first exposure to their domain between the ages of three and eight. Giving them adequate time to develop in their domain and explore their arenas, getting to know them thoroughly. A parents' costs for something like this, say for a national level swimmer, was estimated by Chambliss to exceed $5,000 per year in 1988, with inflation, it's much higher now. To be clear, you don't need to be a master at everything. Just one thing. If you can **master how to learn, how to practice, your life will be extraordinary.**

<u>Concentration | Feel the Mistake | Feel the Way</u>

If you have read this far, you know something about concentrating. To read word after word, sentence after sentence and page after page, took concentration. You couldn't just skip over words and absorb the material. You had to focus. This took energy and can be mentally exhausting. Playing music as we know takes a lot of concentration.

Let's say you're playing the guitar. It's out of tune. We know this because when we pluck the cord, it sounds twangy. It doesn't match the harmonics of the song played before. How do we fix this? We turn the tuning pegs at the end of the guitar, pluck and twist until it gets into the proper pitch. That plucking and twisting is what is called feeling the mistake until you feel the way.

Say the guitar is tuned. You're playing a song. While playing, you miss a chord or don't press hard enough on the string. You can sense the error audibly. By playing that section again, you hear the same mistake. You make a correction. You get closer. You make another until you get closer. **You find the way by feeling the way.** To find the way, you have to concentrate on what sound is coming from the instrument. Your body is the same way. Your body is an instrument. When things are not going the way you need them to, you slow down. Break up the process of what you're doing into steps. Then you identify the mistake and work on it, trying different approaches until you find the way. Then you do it again real time, all together. You may need to add something or take something away from your routine, your diet, your program.

Sleep: The Secret to Performance

The best way to improve after practice is sleep. The best in any sport, sleep more and have better quality sleep than those who don't perform as well. This goes for athletes, writers and students. Pro athletes like Venus Williams and LeBron James average more than 10 hours of sleep a night.

No you can not sleep off your accumulated sleep debt on the weekends and yes, some people can sleep less and still perform. There is a mutation in a gene that is very rare called the DEC2 and less than 1 percent of the population has it. Before you call it a night though, let's go over how NREM and REM sleep improve performance.

NREM and REM

In 1952 at the University of Chicago, Eugene Aserinsky and his professor Nathaniel Kleitman had been studying the eye movement patterns of human infants during the day and night. While monitoring the infant's brain waves, Aserinsky noticed during certain times the infants eyes would move from side to side very rapidly beneath their eyelids, that corresponded with active brain waves. At other times their eyes would be calm and still, again corresponding with brain waves slowly ticking up-and-down. He began to notice a pattern over the nights. His Professor wanted to repeat this study to see if there was any validity. Aserinsky chose his daughter and what they found held true.

They just discovered that we don't just sleep but cycle through two types of sleep every ninety minutes.

- NREM (Non-Rapid Eye Movement)
- REM (Rapid Eye Movement)

What the scientists discovered was that the brain activity of REM sleep was identical to when we were awake and is connected to the experience we know as dreaming. Later NREM sleep was observed and divided up into four stages known as stage 1-4. Here is a brief of what goes on in each stage.

Stage 1 (NREM; Non-REM Sleep)

- In between awake and asleep (twilight zone)
- Light sleep

Stage 2

- Disengaged from surroundings
- Heart rate and respiratory rate are regular
- Body temperature drops below normal range
- Sleep spindles occur

Stage 3 and 4

- Deepest stages of NREM
- Removes unnecessary neural connections aka pruning
- Glial cells clear out neural waste called tau
- Increased blood flow to muscles
- Surges of growth hormone are released as well as other hormones essential for muscle and brain development
- Adenosine is restored aka energy sources
- Tissue growth and repair occurs

Stage 5 (REM)

- Dreams occur
- Brain becomes more active
- Information is synthesized (often in novel ways)
- Neural connections are strengthened
- Body relaxes deeper
- Lowest amount of glucose utilization

Without sufficient amounts of sleep, a waste product known as beta amyloid protein or tau builds up in the deep regions of the brain, particularly in the regions that generate sleep. One area is in the frontal lobes just above the eyebrows or "third eye" area. This is where deep NREM sleep waves are generated. Once build up occurs, sleep quality deteriorates, leaving us more tired, less able to remember and consolidate memories and thus learn and perform at our best. For those of you on a field, in a pool or just trying to make progress in the gym, there are a few studies I'd like to leave with you to think about.

Related to heart health, a study performed to find the effects of insufficient sleep on blood pressure in people doing extensive overtime work in males aged 23-48 years old found one night of sleep reduction of just 1-2 hours significantly increased systolic blood pressure the next day while doing the same or less activity at work. An increase for a day isn't a big deal. Do that for the length of a career and you may lose your life because of it. All because of lack of sleep.

Another study done at the University of Chicago studied five hundred healthy middle aged adults. They tracked the health of the coronary arteries of these individuals as well as their sleep patterns for several years. Over a period of five years the subjects that slept just five to six hours a night or less were 200 to 300% more likely to experience calcification of the coronary arteries (hardening of the vessels) compared to those who slept seven to eight hours a night.

One other reason lack of sleep destroys the body is because of an overactive sympathetic nervous system. The sympathetic nervous system, also known as our fight or flight system, regulates our stress response. In healthy individuals it's activity is short in duration. Only coming on when needed to perform under stress. For example, run from a predator or fight. When this response stays on though, it begins to erode our physiology. One of the chemicals that is released during the stress response is cortisol. It's what is known as a catabolic hormone. Catabolic, meaning breaking down of larger molecules to smaller molecules. Cortisol constricts blood vessels and when this is done over a long period of time, blood pressure remains high, increasing chances of heart attack. High cortisol also breaks down muscle tissue and strains the organs like our liver that recycle hormones.

In relation to sleep, high cortisol also suppresses growth hormone, the holy grail of healing hormones. The Journal of Pediatrics has found that in men approximately 70% of growth hormone pulses occur during stage 3 of NREM sleep. By missing this stage or only getting a partial amount of it makes recovery slower, if it happens at all and if recovery cannot happen muscles won't repair, blood vessels won't repair, and our bones and immune system are compromised leaving us vulnerable to disease. When sleep is sufficient though, NREM sends calming signals to our sympathetic nervous system, reducing our blood pressure, promoting growth hormone release and thus recovery of brain and body tissues.

When it comes to fueling your body for workouts, for performance in school or at work, sleep plays a major role in influencing the choices you make. A study done by Dr. Eve Van Cauter at the University of Chicago conducted research between sleep and appetite.[45] What she found was interesting. She had a series of experiments using healthy adults of normal weight to see if this short sleep was enough to disrupt levels of leptin, ghrelin or both. Leptin is our satiation hormone and tells us that we are full. Ghrelin is our hunger hormone and increases our appetite.

In the first series of five nights each participant got an eight hour sleep opportunity. The second series of five nights each participant got a five to six hour sleep opportunity. Each participant was given their own room, bed, and access to television and Internet. The only thing they couldn't have was caffeine.

In both parts of the study participants received exactly the same amount and type of food and physical activity remained the same. She discovered that when these individuals slept four to five hours a night, despite being given the same amount of food and being similarly active, they were hungrier and had more cravings than when they slept eight or more hours a night.

One more study was conducted with one added element. Fit and healthy individuals went through four nights of eight and a half hours of sleep and then went through four nights of four and a half hours of sleep. On the last day of the experiment the individuals were offered an additional food buffet for four hours after lunch. In the buffet was meats, vegetables, bread, potatoes, salad and fruit as well as ice cream. In the snack bar there was an array of junk foods like cookies and chocolates. Each subject was asked to eat alone to limit social influences.

Even with consuming close to 2,000 calories during lunch, the sleep deprived individuals went in on the snack bar. On average they consumed an additional 330 calories from the snack bar compared to when they were getting eight hours of sleep. Dr. Van Cauter found that cravings for sweets increased by 30 to 40%. While cravings for protein rich foods like meat and fish increased only by about 10% to 15%.

Sleep researcher Dr. Matthew Walker after hearing of Dr. Van Carter's study decided to conduct his own research on why we choose particular food items. Why would someone choose doughnuts over leafy green, knowing what would benefit their performance long-term? He had healthy, average weight individuals engage in a full night of sleep and one sleep deprived night. In each circumstance they were asked to view eighty similar food images. All the images consisted of fruits and vegetables like strawberries, apples and carrots as well as refined high calorie foods such as ice cream and doughnuts.

In comparing the patterns of brain activity while the participants were fully rested and sleep deprived they discovered that the regions of the prefrontal cortex, the area of our brain where we make rational decisions, had become less active by insufficient sleep. Areas of the limbic system and brainstem were amplified in response to the food images. For this reason, high calorie foods became more desirable in the eyes of people who had insufficient sleep. Instead of allowing the participants to engage in actually eating the food of their desires, they just picked out what images they craved the most. When they counted up the extra food items the participants craved it added up to more than 600 extra calories in their daily diet.

Not only does sufficient sleep control hedonistic desires but it also restores and maintains a healthy microbiome. This is because our gut nervous system known as our enteric nervous system is intimately connected with our sympathetic nervous system. Our sympathetic nervous system is intimately connected to our limbic system, the emotional center of our brain. So when the sympathetic nervous system is in balance so is our gut.

In a study done in 2015 involving 10 healthy young men, researchers had them spend eleven days in the laboratory for three-nights of 10-hour bedtimes followed by eight nights of five-hour bedtimes. They discovered **testosterone decreased by as much as 10-15% in men who slept 5 hours or less compared to those who rested.**[47] With lower testosterone, muscle mass decreases and building it back becomes harder. Lack of sleep can lower testosterone levels to that of someone ten years older and having this hormone is critical for performance of athletes and anyone in manual labor jobs.

In a similar study by the University of Chicago, for determining the effects of insufficient sleep on weight loss, researchers had participants stay twice over the period of a month.[49] Once for 14 days in the lab with an 8.5-hour period set aside for sleep. Then once more for 14 days with only 5.5 hours of sleep. They spent their waking hours engaged in home or office-like work activities.

In the full sleep opportunity, each participant slept an average of 7 hours and 25 minutes each night. In the short sleep opportunity, they slept 5 hours and 14 minutes, more than two hours less than in the first part of the study. The number of calories they consumed was about 1,450 per day for each phase.

The average weight loss was surprisingly the same. The difference is in the details though. The participants lost an average of 6.6 pounds during each of the 14 days. During the first phase with adequate sleep, they lost 3.1 pounds of fat and 3.3 pounds of fat-free body mass or muscle. During the short-sleep weeks though, participants lost an average of 1.3 pounds of fat and 5.3 pounds of fat-free mass. Even though the calories were low for the study, that still means by sleeping less and doing the same level of activity and fueling the same way, they stored almost three times more fat and lost almost three times more muscle, just over a period of two weeks. If that doesn't get you to sleep more, this study might.

Chinese researcher Mei-mei Liu and colleagues conducted research on sleep deprivation and sperm health.[50] They used 981 adult men ages 18-50 and divided them into three groups of A, B and C. Each letter denoting a bedtime. Group A went to bed at 8–10 pm, Group B went to bed after 10 pm, and Group C went to bed after midnight. They further divided them into groups of men who slept 6 or less hours, 7-8 hours and 9 or more hours. They found that the groups who slept 6 hours or less and more than 9 hours a night had lower sperm count, less sperm motility and lower survival rates than the group who slept a quality 7-8 hours a night meaning no distractions or wakings. They also found elevated levels of an enzyme known as antisperm antibody or ASA in samples of ejaculate collected. ASA are immune reactive agents produced by the body as a response against the proteins contained in spermatozoa, destroying the body of the sperm and thus its ability to stay motile and fertilize an egg. In short, regular short sleep and regular long sleep makes for poor swimmers in and out of the pool, gentlemen.

Sleep Spindles and Learning

In the areas of any field, be it in the sciences or that of a literal field, memory and piecing learned information together in creative ways is critical to the growth of oneself and organization. Sleep does just that.

After a lecture that Matthew Walker had given, a pianist walked up to him to thank him for his presentation.[51] The pianist went on to describe an experience he has very often which is practicing a particular piece of music in the late evening, getting close to mastering it but yet still missing the mark. He would make the same mistake over and over again in the same particular place or in a particular movement. He would then go to bed and try again the next morning and when he did he could just play the piece smoothly.

After speaking with this pianist, Dr. Walker was inspired to do more research on how this may happen and could become a conscious way of practicing. He took a group of right handed individuals and had them learn to type a number sequence on a keyboard with their left hand as quickly and as accurately as they possibly could. One group learned in the morning and the other learned in the evening. He had them do this for 12 minutes, taking a short break in between each practice. Each participant improved by the end of the 12 minutes. Once this was done they were tested again 12 hours later. The group that had learned the sequence in the morning were tested later that evening after remaining awake across the day. The evening group practiced then was allowed an 8-hour sleep opportunity plus an additional four hour delay to make a 12-hour total rest period like the first group. Those that remained awake across the 12 hours showed no evidence of improvement in performance. Those who slept eight hours showed a 20% jump in performance speed and a 35% improvement in accuracy of the new learned sequence.

What was causing this effect?

In a study to find out how sleep refreshes our ability to make short term memories to long term memories, Dr. Walker began testing people's memory using daytime naps. He recruited healthy adults and divided them into groups of napping or no napping. At noon on the first day of the study, they went through a session of learning one hundred face name pairs with the intention of overloading their short term memory area in the brain, the hippocampus. After learning the name face pairs, the nap group napped for ninety minutes while hooked up to an EEG machine to measure brain wave activity. The next group stayed awake in the lab and performed simple activities such as playing board games. At 6 pm that evening the recruits performed another round of one hundred face name pairs. They found that those who stayed awake became progressively worse at learning or memorizing the names to faces although their ability to concentrate remained stable. Those who napped did much better, **improving their capacity to memorize facts by 20% compared to the no mapping group.**

The reason for this? Sleep spindles.

Sleep spindles are created in stage 2 of NREM sleep. They are fast bursts of brainwave activity at the end of each individual slow wave of NREM sleep. Sleep spindles occur both during deep sleep and in the later lighter stages of NREM sleep. They help to keep an individual asleep, keeping them more resilient to external noise that would potentially wake them up, which would disturb the workings of the brain. Dr. Walker found that the more sleep spindles a participant had during their nap in the study above, the greater their capacity of learning was when they woke up. This is what the pianist was experiencing when he could wake up the next day, and play the part he was making errors on the evening before.

After participants had slept, Dr. Walker could see where the memories had gone using an fMRI. The different parts of the brain regions lit up in the scanner showing where activity had shifted. He noticed that the new motor memories had been shifted to brain circuits that operate below the level of our consciousness meaning they are now second nature. This type of learning is the goal of elite level coaching and elite level performers. In fact, in 2015, the International Olympic Committee stated the critical importance and essential need for sleep in athletic development across all sports for men and women.[52]

With this information now at hand, give yourself a 8-hour sleep opportunity every night. Once you start to sleep better and practice smarter, your performance will improve and you will begin winning more in your life.

Summary of Practice

$$E [QR + C(T) + FbM + AR + N = DR]$$

This equation sums up habit and practice. It means **within an environment** conducive to practice one who performs **quality repetitions** plus **consistency** multiplied by **time** plus **feedback from a Master** plus **adequate rest** plus **nutrition** equals **desired results**. Quality reps have to take place to form skills, consistency produces a stimulus for the myelin and skills to develop, compounding over time getting faster and faster in shorter amounts of time so long as there is accurate, adequate feedback. Adequate rest grows the circuits and myelin and preserves the circuits. Nutrition being both physical and visual fuels the process leading to the desired result.

> "With your spirit settled, accumulate practice day by day and hour by hour. Polish the twofold spirit, heart and mind. Sharpen the twofold gaze, perception and sight."
> —Miyamoto Musashi

On Philosophy

What is Philosophy? Philosophy is simply a way of living. It's a combination of living what we learn and learning as we live. It's how we conduct ourselves in our daily lives alone and with others.

Philosophy is often portrayed as some banal, lecture course. Almost like a dry Sunday school class with a monotone teacher and as much as writing and talking about philosophy is important, it's only the tip of the iceberg. The ancients saw philosophy differently and even when they did write down what they believed, they read it aloud and practiced it with each other.

The written words here are to communicate more effectively across space and time. We only experience the writing here by having lived the experience or are already living them now. Experiment with these texts above and below by living that way and finding out if these are truths for you. A great sage once said, "if that which is true does not work, it is false. If that which is false works, it is true. This may only be for you, in your reality, your world but that which is your reality, even false for another, may be true for you."

> "Most people imagine that philosophy consists in delivering discourses from the heights of a chair, and in giving classes based on texts. But what these people utterly miss is the uninterrupted philosophy which we see being practiced every day in a way which is perfectly equal to itself... Socrates did not set up grandstands for his audience and did not sit upon a professorial chair; he had no fixed timetable for talking or walking with his friends. Rather, he did philosophy sometimes by joking with them, or by drinking or going to war or to the market with

them, and finally by going to prison and drinking poison. He was the first to show that at all times and in every place, in everything that happens to us, daily life gives us the opportunity to do philosophy."
— Plutarch

Just by simply living out our day to day lives, we each share a particular philosophy. One in which provides pleasure, pain, knowledge or understanding or sometimes all of them together. Nonetheless, our philosophies are a guide to how we conduct ourselves in a particular environment everyday. The Greeks had many types of philosophies. A few were *Philoposia*, the joy and interest one takes in drinking. *Philotimia*, the inclination to obtain honors and prestige and the one we are centrally focused on here, *Philosophia*, the interest one takes in wisdom.

It may seem obvious but some of us do not know where or how to begin to find a philosophy or their philosophy to govern themselves or their activities. **Philosophy begins by asking questions.** Socrates once said "the unexamined life is not worth living." What he meant, I believe was, we have to look at our life and ask the hard questions. Hard questions open doors to what we don't know. The things we don't know, hold the greatest gifts.

How?

Jordan Peterson, a renowned psychologist answers this question well: "The unrealized world manifests itself when we make errors and the unrealized world is something that can bring us down but it is also the source of all new information. It's an infinite source of information. In short, as long as what we are doing is working then we know enough. As soon as whatever we're doing stops working, that's instant evidence that there's something about us that needs to be updated."

We only find out about the world by staying curious, asking the hard questions, examining our actions and testing our beliefs against what is presenting itself as truth. This philosophy of living an examined life, asking questions, will often provoke deep feelings and more often than not be uncomfortable. You're stirring the settled water and mixing up the sediment of your current reality. Things will be clouded for a moment. That's okay. It's part of the process. It's a reorganization of who you may believe you are. Once the dust clears and settles back into a new place, what's left is still you. Which is the clarity. Where things were before and where they are now are not who we are, just where we are. We are the witness, the one conscious of all that is going on.

As much as that process can be disturbing and discomforting, it's benefits on the backend propel us into more of our potential. It's like exercise. It burns when we do many reps, it hurts to stretch a muscle a little further than the normal range and our minds and lives are no different. After we're done training, finished stretching, endorphins and blood rush to those areas to bring a natural high and nourish our body. In relating this to life, when we ask properly and confront our beliefs, knowledge and wisdom about ourselves and the world comes into bring about understanding of what, where and who we are.

Now, this does not mean by asking questions that things just open up to you immediately or at all. Some questions will remain unknown. Life is full of mysteries and it's not our responsibility to know everything about everything. What is our responsibility is to know and understand as much as we can. The central idea is becoming self-aware. Aware of our thoughts, actions and results now and their effects in the future. Sometimes we only need to know something once, twice, a few times to move up, to get ahead to the next step in our journey. Then we leave it, making room for the next idea, the next item in our tool bag. These asking questions, using our logic and emotions, are tools. They are to serve us. We are the masters. Use them well.

> "Be patient toward all that is unsolved in your
> heart and try to love the questions themselves,
> like locked rooms and like books written in a
> very foreign tongue, do not now seek the answers,
> which cannot be given to you because you would
> not be able to live them and the point is, to live

everything. Live the question now. Perhaps you
will then gradually, without noticing it, live along
some distant day into the answer."[55]
—Rainer Maria Rilke

What are these hard questions and examinations I'm talking about? They pertain to the places you are not flourishing in but could be or that you want to be but are not. As we have said before, wanting and desiring are irrelevant without action towards the thing we want or desire.

So if your in that boat, you have to ask questions such as:

Why am I not winning?

Why am I not in shape?

Why, in one of the wealthiest countries in the world, am I not wealthy?

Why don't I know more? How can I learn more?

How am I responsible?

How did I get here? How do I go up from here?

How did I contribute to this situation?

Where can I improve? Where did I falter?

Where am I weak? Where am I strong?

What are my deficiencies? Where am I fulfilled?

Where am I headed if I stay on this path?

Who can I reach out to? Who has been here before and lost? Who has won and why?

Was there any luck? Could it be practically repeated?

Am I doing all that I could?

If you notice, it's not all focused on fault but where you are. It's not good or bad until we assign it value but we have an intrinsic idea of what we need to do and where we should be. I encourage you to look in the mirror and ask these questions or sit with yourself with a pencil and notebook and ask these questions as thoroughly as possible. Only you will see these entries. It's for personal insight and only you need to know. Once you know, your life can take a positive direction and the consciousness you bring around others will positively impact them as well, more than likely, without them knowing why or how and that's not important, not central. What's central is the transformation of minds, bodies and spirits.

When we do this type of thinking or mental exercise, we see that more often than not, we are our own barrier even when something stands in our way. What I mean is, though an obstacle is on our path it's up to us to go around, use it or go another way or even through the obstacle. The devil isn't a creature with a forked tongue and a pitch fork. "He" is the obstacles and hindrances we create for ourselves. As much an obstacle is an issue, we don't control that. We can control our actions though.

> "The obstacle is the way."
> —Ryan Holiday

We will never rid ourselves of these obstacles either. Machiavelli writes in *Discourses*, Book 1, Chapter 6: "If one looks carefully, this pattern can be observed in all human affairs: one can never remove one problem without another one's arising." Buddha said "life is suffering." So long as we are alive we will be faced with obstacles, setbacks and disappointments. Wisdom exists in disciplining our disappointments. Grieving, then using the information. Recognizing the treasure in the setbacks and choosing the obstacle of lesser friction.

Inner Change Before Outer Awareness

In what is called Panchatantra, Indian fables about animals, there is a story of a mouse and magician. This Mouse, like most mice, was afraid of cats. He was always in fear and feeling anxiety of a cat. One day a magician, thinking it helpful, transformed the mouse into a cat. Each of them thinking that by becoming the object of fear itself the fear would subside. The fear would be known. So they changed the outward appearance but the mouse within the cat now became afraid of a dog. The fear remained the same. Only the outward appearance changed. The trembling remained. Next the magician changed the cat into a dog. Now the dog was afraid of a tiger. He then turned the dog into a tiger and the tiger was afraid of the Hunter. Finally the magician said to the mouse "I'm going to change you back to your original state because I can change your bodies but I cannot change you. With the heart of a mouse, the fear will remain."

When we change only the outside, gathering things or moving places, but do not first seek to evaluate and change our values that hold us back, we keep getting the same result.

"The world is revealed through the template of your values. When the world you are seeing is not the world you want, it's time to examine your values. It's time to rid yourself of your current presuppositions. It's time to let go of who you are for who you could become."
—Jordan B. Peterson

In the story above, it's not just looking like a tiger but obtaining the heart of a tiger. Which translates to becoming a character of strength, depth and solidity, decisiveness, confidence and power.

"Everywhere I go, there I am."
—Unknown

The Set of The Sail

In Cub Scouts they have an event called the Raingutter Regatta. As fancy as that sounds it was quite simple. We were given kits to build miniature sailboats. We could build them just about any way we wanted to, along the lines of the organization's rules, basically as it comes in the box, no added performance enhancements (we did have one with flame decals though and that probably helped.) We sailed across a large PVC pipe that was cut in half capped at both ends filled with water.

The trick was to hit the wooden mast of the hard plastic sail in the center as you blew the sailboat, with the sail not too taught but not loose either. Then as we walked beside the rain gutter, to keep our eyes on the next few inches to go and ignore the background of the audience. As easy as that sounds, not all the boats sat in the water level. If you blew too low on the sail the nose could pop up, blew too high the nose would dip forward or if you blew too hard it could tip over.

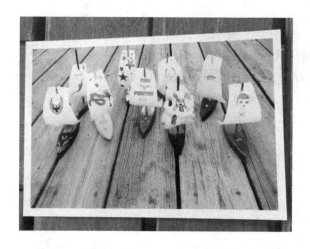

I believe our life is just like a sailboat and having our sail set for where we desire to go determines where we arrive. The same breath could blow upon the sailboat but if the sail isn't set right, it won't go very far. Jim Rohn stated well in one of his self development seminars that "In life, the same wind blows on us all. The wind of adversity, the wind of pain, the wind of loss, the wind of failure. The difference is what we do about it." It's how we set our sail, our mindset and then with that mindset, acting to change our circumstances for the better. It's not what happens to us but what we do about it. Setting the sail is akin to using adversity to propel us forward. It's fuel. The winds of the world will batter those who don't have their sail set in the right position. Those who do, who's mindset is strong and positive will be able to guide themselves in the storms of life and across the choppy waters of adversity.

One of the kids' parents that participated in the cub scouts with us actually would sail. He enjoyed this past time with friends and also with drinks. One day he went out sailing with a friend and they both were drinking, not wearing life vests. The wind picked up and this man slipped and fell from the boat. He couldn't get back in and his friend couldn't get him either because he was too intoxicated.

He drowned. He left a family behind. He set his sailboats sail but forgot to set his own. His mindset was in the wrong place and it cost him his life.

Philosophy as stated above will vary from person to person. It will work well or poorly according to the environment, the culture, the times or era in which one is living and even gender or age. The key is to adopt a mindset that makes situations better, not worse. On average that's going to be operating out of a positive mindset. In fact, it's been shown that positive thinking improves performance by 31% over negative thinking. At times, will you have to be negative, sure. Negative is normal. Some things are negative. It's part of life and to root it out is to uproot ourselves. Sad things should make us sad but we don't live there. We feel and then need to move on. We need to remember and then move forward with the experience in our treasure trove of wisdom. Adopt a philosophy that not only gets you wins while you're here but one that you'd be proud to leave with your children, grandchildren and their children with and beyond them so they, too, can have a model and know how to set their sail when the tides get high and the winds picks up, because they will.

On Love

> Love is the meaning of Life.
> — Osho

From babies to men, from women to animals, even those who don't speak our language, each speaks and knows what love is. Endless battles and sieges have been fought because of it. Blood spilled in the name of love. Children are in a sense born out of it, as well as our own personal inanimate creations into which we breathe life. Relationships are formed and bonded through love. Love knows no time, it is timeless. Love knows no distance, it's infinite. In short, Love is powerful.

Before I go any further I'd like to point out anything you see written here on love will be false insofar as love cannot be written nor can it be intellectualized, as in thought about then called love. "About" means knowing something through someone else's experience or knowledge and love is a state of being, love is primal. We have to experience it to know it for ourselves. We have words to describe it but it is not the words itself. It is in the feeling of a lived experience. Just as you can explain and think about how to ride a bike, it's never actually riding a bike and even if you've never actually rode one before you can still know all about it. How it works and all it's specs. Until you've had to find your balance and go up hills and down hills, pump the brakes and navigate terrain, you won't know biking. And everyone's experience of love is different, though there are great similarities. Not that that's bad, it's just different. There's nuances to everything. Someone else's nuance may spark new feelings of understanding in you.

Personally I've been fortunate to have found and cultivated a true romantic love twice in my life. Each opened up a new avenue of creativity and strength and also a new depth of sorrow. I was cultivating new levels of awareness.

Though in each case coming on like a raging fire with the first relationship and just as passionate in the second, it slowly simmered down and the relationship went in a new direction. At the time, not the direction I wanted it to, but as cliche as it sounds, looking back, it was what I needed. I was given the opportunity to look myself in the mirror and ask myself the tough questions:

- What choice did I make to cause this?
- How could it have been handled better?
- What am I not doing or could be doing better?

This is not to say other factors outside of my control weren't present (they always are), but rather I gave myself something to be responsible for and positioned myself for positive change. Simply by being a person, you're worthy of love but when we fail to evoke the responses desired from a beloved or our family, it's time to look at yourself in the mirror, take responsibility for your actions and discover the deficiencies in your actions or possibly your character. We are all imperfect and faulted, but that doesn't mean we are destined to stay that way. So don't stop there.

We can find a model, we can find couples winning. If they are friends, observe them. If they are in books, read about them. Remember, certain ways of speaking and behaving create feelings in you and evoke feelings and responses from others. Three books in particular, made clear to me what the key elements are and I'll cover them for both men and women.

They are:

- A Man's Guide to Women
- Love and Respect
- Deeper Dating

Each will be briefly discussed below. I've extracted key elements that may be of use to you as they have been of great utility in my life.

<u>Types of Love</u>

When thinking of love what comes to mind? The movie, The Notebook? Paris and the Eiffel Tower? Valentine's

Day? I'd imagine they more often invoke images of living things like people or pets.

Each of those items above, days or places merely symbolizing love, particularly romantic love, are only part of the types of love there are. There is familial love or brotherly love; love of family and kin or those like family or kin. Communal love; love of community and town and the one most of us know and is the most sought after, romantic love; passion and affection with intimate actions associated with the relationship.

What do these and all forms of love have in common?

You.

They stem from you. Some people and activities are easy to love. We get along well, we have a natural inclination toward them. Others we don't and over time we may learn to respect and appreciate our differences and may learn to love the challenges these people or activities bring. Nonetheless though, love in all its forms comes from us.

Now that may sound obvious but what about that girl you loved who left? How did you feel about it? That guy who broke your heart? Or the parent or leader who let you down?

I can imagine that at that moment you forgot the love came from you, that you created it through associated thoughts and chemicals in your body. I know I didn't the first couple times. That same person who you loved could walk by another person and not cause that response of love like it has in you and before they came into your life, love was there possibly for some other romantic partner or the other parent or leader. So was it something they gave you or was it something they helped evoke out of you, that was already there but like a lock needed a code with just another number in it to open you up?

I encourage you to find what love is for you. How do you define love?

For me, Love is an expression of lasting affection, gratitude and attention to a person or activity that provides the giver and receiver with pleasure and joy. It's an unconditional positive regard for the best in yourself and those around you. It can endure almost any "how" with a great enough purpose. It's nonjudgmental, yet holds you and others to higher standards and understands your struggles and doesn't shutter from them. It makes one stronger and more resilient in all ways. Love is something that comes from labor and working towards enhancing your own life as well as one another's or many people's lives. It heals and sometimes hurts but it's pain is that of growth.

In the Family

This is where love begins. It's where we are shown and learn how to be loved and love ourselves. Parents or a parent, or a guardian show us, through how they treat themselves and how they treat others, what level of love and kindness is appropriate in different areas of life. If you have siblings you may know what I mean. As kids, we often think the world revolves around us because in one sense it does. People tend to our needs, our wants, and our calls for attention. We intrinsically know that attention equals affection. When siblings also get the same or more attention it feels as if we are being displaced. We're not in the grand scheme of things but we are learning how to be patient, we learn we aren't the central point and that giving our attention to those less developed than us can help them grow and by helping them we also grow. The store or the market can be chaotic, little ones may cry for something they want. As we mature, we begin to pick up on signals that it's time to step up and help our parent or guardian, that by soothing the one in distress we get to have peace now and likely peace later. We may not call it love then but we understand that by giving our attention and affection to our family member in need, greater rewards than toys and gadgets come our way in the form of freedom and respect.

That's a simple example but it's not always that smooth and it takes an enormous amount of time to achieve that in kids. Reasoning with someone under ten years old who's hungry and tired is like trying to herd cats. It doesn't work well. You're better off putting the food down and making the environment loving and easy to maneuver in so that the both of you or group of you can operate smoothly. What's great about family though, is they are permanent. They are with us for life. When we fail, we get the opportunity to try again with them. We get to learn patterns of behavior and how to handle it better to get our way or just the result needed. When we are young, we have to be together, we learn to work together because we have to if we are to stay sane and maximize our growth. We learn to give our sister space so she will be charged up after dinner to play games or give our brother a hand with chores so we can get out in the yard faster and play longer. In that process our siblings may poke and prod and joke but that too is helping to strengthen us. They do it sometimes to inflict pain but on a deeper level, it's to help make us resilient in life. Without that early teasing or pressure, life still comes by to offer it to us in much harsher ways later. If we didn't build resilience when we were younger with love behind the hard times it's unlikely we will fare well when it comes as an adult.

In the family is also the place where we can be authentic in our expressions. Anger, sadness, fear and joy as well as many other emotions can be expressed and even when we are wrong for acting a certain way, forgiveness is often not far away. Our families know things about us that sometimes we forget or don't know about ourselves and can remind us of who we are and where we are going. They keep us going when we falter. One of the other great things about family is the intermingling of people. Say mom's side is very rugged, working class, and knows some of the unwritten laws of the world and dad's side comes from education, military and financial success. It's highly unlikely that these people would be together on a regular basis in the year other than the fact that your parents came together as a family unit. We get a wealth of wisdom from each side. The youngest of the family can sit with someone who's in their eighties and discuss the latest sports or banter about relationships formed in school or how to solve problems they are currently having. We discover parts of life that we haven't lived into and it prepares us for the upcoming years or we get reminded of where we have come from and are able to pass down our hard won wisdom to a younger niece or nephew to help them better navigate their situation.

Love is so valuable because in the world it's not so common. The average stranger won't give you a chance, let alone a second chance and they are likely interested in you for themselves rather than your well-being. The warm tender hand of love we know from loved ones is a blessing. It is not the norm. The world is indifferent to us and the attention we receive from family and close friends in the community is to be cherished and revered.

In the Community

On a larger scale, the community and towns we live in can also offer love, a sense of security and support. Not all communities are like this and that's what makes the ones that are unique and sought after. I live in one and the effects of being here on my life, I believe are better because of it. Like in a family of blood relation, a communal family offers a diverse perspective and eclectic sort of knowledge we don't always get in school or from our immediate circle. We find these unique people in the grocery stores, the gym, the restaurants, the school or in activity clubs. They provide a reason to get out of our place of comfort and explore the world. When times are tough, they often lend a helping hand in the form of wisdom or home cooked meals or the literal hand of moving furniture or the building of a new project. In being in the community we learn about different cultures and how they live, where they come from and understand and relate to their story. We in essence connect to a greater consciousness around us. Our shared insights are able to benefit more than just the sum of our families.

Self-Love

> "It's dark, yet illuminated within; it's a path you travel alone, yet you carry within all those you care for; it leads to nowhere and everything...it's our existence, it's love."
> —Ricardo M. Yslas

This is a topic that many people know yet neglect. Those that participate, particularly men are looked down upon. Why? Because love is often viewed as something soft, warm and fuzzy. Yet there's also tough love. Discipline is a form of self love. It's not all about massage, relaxation and vacation. Though if you have been working like your life depended on it then it might entail those items.

Self love, I believe, is bestowing those things you need upon yourself even if it means slowing down a bit and stepping back. Remember, we are in life for the long haul, not just the weekend meatheads and that goes for you too ladies. Notice I said <u>need</u>. What do I mean by need?

- Real Food
- Shelter
- Clean Water
- Clean Air
- Rest

Everything else is a want. You don't need new clothes if the ones you have fit and are season appropriate. You don't need to go out for dinner if you just bought groceries. You don't need the newest things to improve your quality of living. Yes, it feels good to have new things. Yes, some new technology does improve the quality of our lives but just striving to get the new when we can use what we have without straining ourselves is more optimal. If you have the financial means then do it but that also means you likely have been bestowing upon yourself the money to do so. You were disciplined and earned it. What really improves the quality of our life after we have taken care of our tangible necessities, is the quality of our thinking. The intangible is also a source of nutrition in our lives. How we speak to ourselves has a massive impact on our performance and confidence. What we ingest visually, mentally and audibly, through books, audio, conversation with others and our environment will determine how we perceive our reality. As we have discussed earlier, how we perceive our reality will determine who we see ourselves as and how we respond to our environment. Our actions will determine how others respond to us and when we respond with love, kindness and compassion, we not only are more likely to receive those virtues in return, we as individuals grow more confident and feel more supported to approach and engage with others in our family, community and with our intimate partner. It's an energizing cycle that spirals upward.

Once we have laid the foundation of having our physical necessities in order, we can then build onto that with our wants in each category. We can improve in each category as we grow and develop ourselves. Some may ask how do we know we are getting the right necessities? Look at yourself. Are you healthy? Are you out of the harsh elements of Nature? Are you hydrated? Are you tired or do you have energy? What state is your mind, body and spirit in?

Then look at those in places who are winning. What are they doing? What are they eating? How are they living? How did they get there? Study them. Ask them directly for their advice. They will more than likely be glad to share with you how they have achieved their standard of living so long as they are not in the middle of a task important to them. More than likely though, you know what you need to do to heal and feel strong and good about yourself. **<u>Do that thing.</u>**

So in this there are two sub groups of Self-Love:

- Warm and Fuzzy love
- Rough and Tough love

Warm and Fuzzy

This type of love is referring to the sensual. It's a massage from a partner or the beach vacation you've been thinking of or just a day off to sleep and recover from the weeks of working. It could be a hot shower and a warm meal with someone you enjoy your time with. However you do this type of relaxing, it is in essence, an activation of our para-sympathetic nervous system. This activation reduces our stress hormones like cortisol and increases feel good neu-rotransmitters like dopamine and serotonin. For those in the throes of passion with a partner, oxytocin is another relaxing hormone associated with things warm and fuzzy. We will cover oxytocin more deeply in a moment.

Rough and Tough

Not the usual idea of love when we think about it but this type is the one that gets things done. It cuts to the core and makes you better able to love and appreciate love when it's bestowed upon you. It's what makes the warm and fuzzy type of love feel good.

An example would be working out. You're in a sense tearing yourself down to build yourself back up later. It's going to make you better and you do it for the benefits of mind and body. It's activating our sympathetic nervous system and bringing about a natural high from the rush of endorphins. If it comes from other people it's usually in the form of criticism. Consider the context and relationship of course before indulging in their critique but if it's from a close friend or family member or your beloved, take notice. They are more than likely looking to help you grow out of the plateau you're living on. They aren't doing it to be a jerk. They are doing it because they see you're capable of more and believe you can handle the flack they are giving you. If they aren't, ignore it. It means nothing and is a false opinion. You know what's true so live that. Soon it will be irrefutable what's true and they will likely come to you for advice and guidance. Just keep taking the next step on your path.

The key is to know when you should be soft and when you should be tough. You discover this knowledge by asking questions. Find where you are and what you really need to do to be in an optimal state. If you are unable to do so, elicit the help of close friends or family. There are also professional people who specialize in guiding people into healthier patterns. Call them. Do whatever it takes to get yourself right because when you do, we without saying, give permission to the next gal or guy to do the same. We set the example.

God only knows what will happen when you put
your house in order. Certainly things that you do
not currently regard as possible will happen.
—Jordan B. Peterson

The best thing you can do to grow
stronger is love yourself.
—Tom Bilyeu

Self love and knowing what you need is a practice. Self love is something we have to carve out time for and cultivate intentionally. Will we do this all the time? No. We forget or go beyond our threshold and redline and we need those in our circle to remind us. I'm certainly still learning to do it and it's something we will never stop learning to do.

When people from the outside put you down or even if you yourself feel unworthy, be aware and acknowledge that feeling is there inside yourself and then remember, **you are love**. Bring that love inward and take a moment to reflect on the love in your life. This begins the healing process. This is where strength begins.

Romantic Love | Love as Meditation

Here life appears vibrant no matter where we are. Life is rich and things flow. We are our best selves in these moments of romance. Time seems to stop. The present is all there is. We have contentment, we feel we have all we need. We forget ourselves and only our partner remains. We are selfless. What does this also resemble? Meditation. Love is a meditation. A natural focusing and awareness of the present. It's why lovers have an effortless flow of conversation, of movement and understanding. In Zen they call it an effortless effort. What is often missed is the arduous efforts beforehand. Working on oneself to become ready to receive that person in that moment. As effortless as love may seem, much effort was required to get there. As mentioned before in the last section, when we take care of ourselves and our needs, and make ourselves abundant, we are able to give love and receive love effortlessly.

Love itself though is spontaneous, it's irrational. We don't always consciously choose our partner. Biology is a powerful force that pulls us in the direction of particular mates. As people I'm sure you have experienced this. If not, check out the book The Red Queen by Matthew Ridley. For you guys out there, females choose you, you don't choose them. And if you do choose them and they accept, it's only because they accepted you. It's like that for almost every animal out there and we are no different. What is different though is the way we court in love. The peacock with it's large and exquisite plumage may dance and shake its literal tail feathers, stags may charge and fight with their antlers and orange guppy fish of Trinidad flash their colors amongst the female schools of fish passing by. We as humans have our own ways of conveying love and attracting mates. At the University of Washington, doctors John and

Julie Gottman studied the communication between couples in the "love lab", after they had been apart for eight hours. He video taped each interaction and watched them talk about pleasurable topics, argue and just discuss the day. He monitored their heart rates, their breathing, their galvanic skin response, and their movements in moments of stress and arousal. He went as far as to code their facial expressions, tone of voice, particular words, gestures and emotions. After seeing them together he interviewed each individual and asked about their relationship. Then after a period of one to three years he saw them again. He and his wife did this experiment for twenty years and over the course of a forty year career they have seen thousands of couples interact. What they found was that <u>the conversation is the relationship.</u> This first part of this is for the guys but just as much as it's helpful to them, ladies you will benefit from it too. Here's what they found the best men did.

The main model is something they call:
A-TT-U-N-E.

A-TT-U-N-E stands for

- Attend
- Turn Towards
- Understand
- Non-defensively Listen
- Empathize

<u>Attend</u>: Give your undivided attention when it is needed. That means if she wants to talk to you, you turn off the phone, turn off the game, and show through your actions that you care about her and what she is saying. No matter what she is saying. Attention equals affection. Attention is how we express love.

<u>Turn Toward</u>: Literally turn toward your partner. Women equate intimacy with conversation that is face-to-face and eye-to-eye. Men connect better shoulder-to-shoulder.

<u>Understand</u>: It doesn't matter what she's saying, have your goal be understanding. You get to understanding by asking questions. Questions direct focus. Whatever you do, don't try to distract her and don't try to fix the problem and don't make jokes about her problems. This is about showing genuine interest and concern about the topic of interest and seeking to understand why what she is saying or doing is important to her.

<u>Non-defensively listen</u>: This is key. Most importantly when what a woman is talking about or is upset about is *you*. Don't react to it. Just listen and then respond in a calm manner when she's done. No one likes to be criticized or feel under attack. Don't interrupt and don't forget that any feelings are facts to the person feeling them. Whether or not you agree with how she's reacting or how she views her reality, her feelings are her current reality in that moment

and that constructs her perspective. Stay calm, confident and in control. Your calmness and confidence will help calm her down.

Empathize: Understanding is intellectual while empathy is emotional. Attempt to feel what she is feeling, regardless of whether in your opinion it has any logic to it. This way you can understand her stance fully.

And the last two elements are:

- Integrity
- Trustworthiness

Meaning you are who you say you are and you do what you say you are going to do. She's looking for you to create containers of safety, both physically and emotionally. The way you create safety in conversation is by deeply listening and being genuinely interested.

In short, asking questions is more attractive than talking. Being interested in this other person is much more important than being interesting to them. It's about the other person in front of you. It comes down to character and from character to consciousness, our state of being. It's who we are as men, as a man, that makes us attractive. The material things are helpful but they are only an abstract representation of who we are, not who we actually are and our mates are viewing that. Become the man you need to be and she will find her way to you as you make your way to her. These steps seem small but they, like atoms, make up the big things.

> "Demonstrations of love are small, compared with
> the great thing that is hidden behind them."
> —Kahlil Gibran

Be vulnerable to the extent she sees you're human and understanding. Reserved and compartmentalized to the point where things don't weigh heavily on you in her presence and detached to the extent negativity and negative situations don't phase you. You are calm, confident and in control of your body and emotions.

The next section is for the ladies and it comes from a book called Love and Respect by Emerson Eggerichs.[60] This book has roots in the Bible and religious texts. Emerson has what he calls C-H-A-I-R-S for how women should treat their husbands and has what's called C-O-U-P-L-E for how men should treat their wives. I'll provide a brief view of C-H-A-I-R-S here. Check out the book for more details. It's really great.

C-H-A-I-R-S stands for:

- Conquest
- Hierarchy
- Authority

- Insight
- Relationship
- Sex

<u>Conquest</u>, this is his desire to work and achieve. Conquering in this sense means breaking barriers and overcoming challenges in the world.

To go a little further what's one of the main questions men ask in conversation with one another to further connect. "What do you do for work?" Most men identify with their work and their skill set. Being a man I know this to be true and other men you may ask may confirm the same thing. In the male psyche there is a desire to provide, to lead and serve other people particularly our women. We feel a deep desire to work for the sake of our family. It's not that we don't want to be around more, we do but in order to create that uninterrupted time with our women and family, work will have to be done first. That's why it's critical it's done young and early in the days before other lives call for us.

The biggest thing we want from our women is their belief in us. It's when things get tough and we're tired that simple words of encouragement, thank you's or just the smile and warm hand of our partner pulls us into the next challenge, pushes us to go a little harder and move a little faster. When we push too far, help reel us in from time to time with simple words of appreciation and thankfulness for our work. When you do, we become much more sensitive to your needs.

Hierarchy represents his desire to protect and provide from a position of dominance. This isn't placing a man above a woman but it is placing a great responsibility upon him. When we love our women and family we are not just willing but in extreme cases, expected to give our lives up for them. Many young men have this innate trait to want to protect and provide. Without proper training and education as well as physical and mental development, men can misinterpret this instinct and become what some women call "controlling." And what many young women want in the way of protection and a provider is also misinterpreted because of lack of education and training and physical and mental development about what the male is doing and why he is doing it. Each individual needs to share themselves with the other to care for one another after learning through guidance and experience. Before we give ourselves to someone we have to be there for ourselves.

We must first fill our cup abundantly. Only then is it possible to give unconditionally without resentment or expectation. Focus on yourself so you may give and fulfill the others needs when that occasion presents itself or you see the opportunity to step up. This means learning about yourself first and then about them, but you will learn about yourself as you learn about them too.

As it says in the Bible:

> "The husband must fulfill his duty to his wife and
> likewise also the wife to her husband. The wife
> does not have authority over her own body, but
> the husband does; and likewise the husband does
> not have authority over his own body
> but the wife does."
> —1 Corinthians 7:34

Again, the only way this is possible is by coming to understand the other side better than we currently know our own. The side you're on is more known. It's your nature. Learn from the other and prosper with one another.

Who is or was the head of your family? Likely if there was two parents of opposite sex, it was your father. Most women don't want that position because they have another calling, that of nurturing and assisting the other members of the family while the father or man provides the means and space for her to do that. And a reminder ladies, if the man you're with is abusing this position, it's not the title or position that's the problem, it's his nature and you will not change that. Not before taking a large amount of abuse in the process in which case you both lose and anyone tied to you gets dragged down as well.

Choose a man with a good willed nature and be rewarded. Don't know how to do that? **Study human nature.** Learn about men and your own desires and why their nature turns you on. Just because you have been with one or several males doesn't mean you know men. You probably keep picking from the same group and just because they look different doesn't mean they are different. Find the experts and the studies. We're not what you think and what you yourself have experienced. Just like you, we have many facets of our being. We may be simpler at times but nonetheless we are diverse in our expressions and communications. When you learn our code, respect our way of operating, we seek to understand yours and work with you, live with you and love you to our fullest.

<u>Authority</u> is his desire to serve and lead with purpose. With authority a man is able to carry out responsibilities with focused intent, without distraction or permission. Some of this is biological with testosterone playing a major factor and some of it is psychological in that a man feels he can go all in when he's not competing for power. Along with authority though needs to be competence. Male or female, to lead effectively knowing what to do and how to do it is a major part of obtaining and using authority. Authority without competence leads to inevitable destruction, dissolution and tyranny.

Should considerations be made about decisions to be made in the relationship? Yes. Should concerns and questions be raised? Absolutely. But when shit hits the fan and things need to be done, who do you call on most often? It's usually your man, your dad, brother or some other strong man to help.

<u>Insights</u> are his ability to naturally want to analyze and counsel. As men, we have a tendency to dissect and see things dispassionately with facts and information rather than with feelings and emotions. Not bad, just different. When it comes to romance though it can cause a world of trouble. We each, as men and women, have insights that only a man or woman could know. It's important that we share each other's knowledge and <u>listen</u>.

Women are trained early for this and again hormones like estrogen make this activity a little smoother than with men but nonetheless we both need to <u>listen</u>. We as men desire for our women to trust our insights as we trust their intuitions and heart, and that behind our calculated analytics and desire to hold counsel is our hearts and lived experiences. Not just some feeling or sensation but facts of having lived, learned, lost and won. When we offer our insights it's our way of helping you get well and get results. Trust each other and let your men share their knowledge ladies. If it doesn't serve you that's another thing. Move on and find the knowledge that does. And if you don't want these insights **just tell him** in a kind way, you need a listener and not a speaker.

<u>Relationship</u> is his way of connecting with you and others, in which case it is usually shoulder-to-shoulder.

What does that mean?

Just what it sounds like. Standing or sitting shoulder to shoulder and being with us in our space. That space could be our room, the garage, the gym, the yard, the car, really anywhere. We don't even need you to do anything. Your presence alone energizes us, motivates us to work harder on our project, push harder in our set and be more engaged with the task in front of us. It sounds odd but it's how our bodies and minds work. Ask most men when they are alone, or particularly when they are about to fight or do something hard what they are thinking of and it's likely you and the family. Not what you have said but you. The image of you and the responsibility they have for making sure they overcome this challenge and come home a victor, even if that challenge is at the gym, a sparring partner in training or getting through traffic. Overcoming it with you or with the thought of you strengthens the relationship and commitment to you. When he asks you to do something shoulder to shoulder he's bringing you into his world and sharing his way. It's like you ladies bringing us around your friends or family for dinner or to shop and talking and telling stories as they size us up for you. Some even have friends that test us. Our shoulder to shoulder is our ritual just as your eye to eye conversations, sharing of emotions and feelings are your rituals. When you are with us, shoulder to shoulder, sharing space and being present, it confirms that you like us, that you care and that is what we need to know.

<u>Sex</u>. We know what that means. The male drive is high for intimate relations with our woman and many times, for a lot of women. Testosterone is one of the hormones that causes this high libido and its natural. Where men fall short is giving the slow affection and building up to sex and where women lack is the not being sensitive to the drive of a man's libido. As a guy, it can be intense. When we love someone, we want to show them and that is usually through physical touching and intercourse. Can we be too quick? Absolutely. It's something we must work on through training our PC muscles and actually moving slower so as to build the passion. Be patient. With that in mind, we as men need to take that into consideration and put you first. Imagine if your man stopped allowing you emotional release for, say a month. You'd be cranky. You'd probably call someone up to get that release wouldn't you? You may even find another partner to give you that emotional release! And I know, sex involves many more elements and possibly lives will come from the act but it's the principle. It's a need for us, just as emotional release is a need for you.

And since this section is for the ladies, if you feel your need isn't being met, give first. I'm not saying get him off first. I'm saying give first. Initiate the first move. Come on to him a little. Stir him up inside. We love to initiate sex with you but when you initiate first, it's incredibly attractive and almost irresistible. Again, like in any relationship, give before you get. If you need more pillow talk, more affection without the sex, tend to his needs then <u>ask for what you want and need</u>. If he doesn't respond and doesn't live up to his word, you have material to build a case and if it's not working still, end the relationship because it was done before it started. And will you be turned down sometimes? Unlikely but a possibility. Just as you don't always want it, he may not either. Respect that. Move into another arena for the time being. Things may heat up there.

<u>More on Sex</u>

I'll keep this simple. Sexual healing is real. The hormones that we produce from engaging in such an act are as good if not better than going to the gym. It lowers blood pressure, engages our core, exercises our legs, increases blood flow and stimulates the mind. It's more than just physical though, there's a bond being formed that will bring two people literally as close as they can get but also link them together when they are apart. This act will potentially bring another life through it that is of each of you. It's sacred and should be treated as such. Is there time for a quick shag with your partner sometimes? Of course. But that's not the regular routine, it's a novelty. Make time for one another. Having our priorities in order as well as ourselves and our spaces in check, we make the act of love much more effortless and enjoyable. We grow in mind, body and spirit when we take our time and savor each moment.

"Just as space is needed for true productivity, slow
and effortless touch is needed for real ecstasy."
—Michael Holt

The key concepts are:

- Practice it safely

- Practice it often

- Participate fully aware

- Go in knowing another life may come of your actions and be ready to take responsibility if it does

- Think of your partner first. Feel their internal energy (Ladies first gentlemen)

- Take your time and go slow. It's not a race, there's no time limit and you should want to linger here with your partner

- Set the environment up for the act (stimulate all five senses)

- Make and hold eye contact

- Make time for conversation or "pillow talk". At a minimum just stay close to your partner. Caress and hold one another.

Essentially in both books I just paraphrased, the essential elements are love each other and respect each other's needs. See where one another is coming from. Step into their position for a moment. **Listen.** Sacrifice for one another and you will each be taken care of. The type of giving and sacrifice will be different for each person but the point is to **give and sacrifice**, love and respect, listen and learn. When we do this for each other, we find our relationship with ourselves and our partner grows and flourishes.

> Your sex is deeply rooted and connected to
> who you are as creator, as a man. It is a force of
> nature, of which you have dominion over, and the
> medium through which you can manifest yourself
> and resources to obtain your aims. It is a gift you
> bestow and evoke from the women in your life and
> through which your children are created and born.
> —Destin Gerek

Love Drugs | Dopamine, Oxytocin and Vasopressin

Oxytocin or the "cuddle hormone" as some call it, is one of the key elements in pair bonding in humans and creating the feelings of love in our lives, particularly romantic love.

Not only is it for partners of the unrelated opposite sex, it plays a role in bonding between mother and child. As warm and cozy oxytocin makes us feel, love has its roots in aggression and our sympathetic nervous system. So let's dive into that for a moment.

What happens when you first encounter the person you are attracted to? For most, the hands sweat, the heart rate and breathing increase and pupils dilate. We are in fight or flight. Adrenaline and cortisol are flooding our vasculature and heightening our senses. We are ready to act, to respond to reach our beloved or possibly run in the face of rejection. This response is short term and shouldn't last throughout a relationship otherwise it would deteriorate our physiology and our mind. In short, this stress response, be it in a fight with an opponent, an encounter with the hot girl in the squat rack or that Clark Kent looking guy in the produce section, the initial stress response is to amplify our initial attraction and pull us near this person, if not at first physically, then at least keep them in mind until we can get close.

The same symptoms of being madly in love are the same symptoms of someone who has gone mad. Symptoms such as anxiety, restlessness, and hypervigilance. We crave the affection and presence of the beloved. The circuitry of our brain, the centers which release reward chemicals, like dopamine are stimulated and active in this state. The same brain regions that light up in love are also stimulated by using the drugs cocaine or amphetamines. The same symptoms of mania, energy and drive are evoked, yet there is a major difference, drugs pull us away rather than draw us in toward one another. Love provides nourishment, protection and healing on the back end that those harmful substances don't. Love is like eating a balanced diet of whole foods. We can have the sweetness of the fruit but with a fiber that balances the absorption of nutrients and provides energy all day. Drugs are like refined food, driving energy up quickly then leaving the consumer crashing and their bodies devoid of nutrients, leading to a spiral downward in health and vitality.

Some people fall prey to those substances and it's not entirely their fault, yet nonetheless they bear the responsibility of the happenings and actions that ensue. The hormone oxytocin may provide a way to get out of that way of living and into a way of being and loving that benefits everyone. The Beatles may have been on to something when they said "All you need is love, love. Love is all you need." It could be all we need to get started on our path to a better way of being.

The Healing Power of Oxytocin

In the Journal of the Society of Neuroscience researchers found that social bonding reduced the rewarding properties of amphetamines through the dopamine D1 receptor mediated mechanism. This translates into simply being engaged with others in a healthy environment can rewire our reward centers that control oxytocin to function optimally in a natural way to bond with others over time. How much time? It varies. We are all wired in different ways and our habits will dictate the depth of our addictions and patterns but as we discussed above, when we change the environment and make it satisfying, as well as easy and obvious we can begin to change.

Heart Meditations are also a way to stimulate the release of oxytocin. By focusing on the heart and from the heart thinking of unconditional love you have given or someone has given you for a period of time, feelings of love will arise. When feelings of love arise, oxytocin is being released, signaling nitric oxide to be produced, a vasodilator meaning opening of the blood vessels. Nitric oxide then signals the chemical called endothelium-derived relaxing factor which cause the arteries in our heart to literally open wider, allowing more blood, oxygen and nutrients to reach it. With more blood flow, oxygen and nutrients become available to our heart and body, our heart and body can begin to heal itself and love will begin in that moment to start to become your state of being.

Like humans, prairie voles are highly social, monogamous rodents that like alcohol (ethanol) and being similar to humans they are thought to be useful in understanding social influences on alcohol (ethanol) consumption. Here's a study done on them regarding the social influences on preventing alcohol consumption.

In the first experiment , the voles were housed in isolation for four weeks with 24 hour access to 10% ethanol in a two-bottle choice test. Researchers then removed the ethanol solution from the cage for 72 hours or 3 days. Animals remained in isolation and were then housed with a unfamiliar same-sex partner to be social with, and ethanol access was allowed again. The voles that remained isolated showed an increase in ethanol intake relative to pre-deprivation baseline, typical of relapse-like behavior. The animals that were socially housed with a familiar same-sex partner did not show an increase in ethanol intake, and this was independent of whether the social partner had access to ethanol as well. As we do more research and experiment, science is beginning to discover that the social affiliations and the oxytocin released from it, may reverse the neuroadaptations occurring with repeated drug and alcohol use. With this information, our future has the potential to be more loving and supportive of those struggling with addiction and abuse.

This goes to show relationships are the ultimate reward, not just for animals but for humans too and within them we reap a bounty of benefits. Some of them are support and camaraderie, laughter and friendship. Another activity associated with this hormone is sex. As stated earlier sexual healing is real. Guess what's released after an orgasm in massive amounts...oxytocin.

Commitment and Love

The prairie vole and the montane vole are virtually the same size, look similar and live in similar environments. What distinguishes the prairie vole from the montane vole is pair bonding. The montane vole is non-monogamous and solitary, while the prairie vole is monogamous and loving.

Why?

Oxytocin and vasopressin. A study done on these cute furry critters revealed that when a female prairie vole found a male vole she was interested in, dopamine spiked and her oxytocin levels increased by 51%. When they inhibited the production of oxytocin by injection of a chemical antagonist, she would lose the loving feelings toward her chosen partner. The male voles were different but similar in that testosterone blocks the effects of oxytocin but responds to vasopressin, a peptide of similar structure and function as oxytocin. When injected with the antagonist to block vasopressin, males lost their loving feelings for their partner.

Now as stated above, females respond to oxytocin and males respond to vasopressin. What this translates into is that women fall in love through sexual intimacy. Men fall in love through commitment. Oxytocin rises in orgasm for women bringing them closer to their partner. They have the receptors for oxytocin readily available. Like most other things, men must earn their receptors.

Men fall in love through being sexually stimulated, though after orgasm vasopressin drops. As we just learned, vasopressin bonds men to their partner. This means men who wait to have orgasms and intercourse with their partner will keep vasopressin elevated while the receptors for oxytocin slowly increase in the brain. Hence why so many women and even men who want to evoke love or feel more loving want to wait to have sex. They know intrinsically that the male brain needs time to catch up to grow more receptors. To grow from lust to love. Thus when the old adages that say men who wait and go slow and don't rush things fall in love, appears to be true. One more element remains, testosterone.

A study done on men in the US Air Force revealed that single men had the highest testosterone, married men and those who are single but committed to a woman had the same levels of testosterone. It may be the reason why older men tell young men to wait to get involved in a committed relationship early. It lowers their testosterone and that may mean lower drive and performance in other areas of life. Yet to trade in some testosterone for true love, appears in nature to be worth it and if you have ever had love, you would also believe that to be true. And so if married men and men committed to a woman but are not married, have the same levels of testosterone that means it's not marriage that men speak of lowering their testosterone, its commitment. You're sacrificing that male element for the treasure of pair bonding, for the higher calling of intimacy and potentially, family.

As wonderful as testosterone is, keeping it high throughout life can cause more bad than good being that it's anabolic and stimulates growth of body tissues. This commitment to our partner and lowering our testosterone may be nature's way of preventing overgrowth, cancer, and other rapid growths that would destroy life. At a minimum, just by having a partner and not feeling isolated improves health. It's been found that isolated men die young, that loneliness increases chances of mortality by 45%.

Being a man myself I know how valuable this hormone testosterone is. I'm not saying give up your testosterone. Cherish it, nurture it and use it to your advantage. But I've been in love and I know it's highs and I know it's low's. Each has its gifts and pains. What's better than feeling hyped up all the time and essentially invincible is having your partner, your woman who loves and supports you through the tough times and the tears. The connection of extended family and the friends and opportunities that brings. Nature and our bodies are wiser than our minds. It may not always be what we want it to be, as in, our bodies may not lead us down our ideal path for our career or into riches and prestige but it's attempting to lead us to the path of more life or children and family, love and longer living. Coupled with our rational mind, we can direct that energy into the virtues of discipline to achieve the award winning career, the big bank account and the social standing that will support our beloved and family for years long after we are gone.

So guys take your time with the ladies you meet, find quality dedicated and supportive women, then listen with your ears and eyes. Ask questions to know what makes their heart sing and what they enjoy and what makes them laugh. Escalate and build tension but hold it, don't break it yet. Let the fire of desire and all its peptides and hormones rise until it spills over and you can pass the reins over to your body, your dark horse and enjoy the moment. After that indulgence and the cascade of rewarding chemicals has flooded your body, continue to court her, in body and word. Keep the conversation alive by learning and reading. The conversation is your relationship.

Ladies, find men who are committed in their life to building themselves and their skills, their business and the lives of others. Listen to what your body craves and before moving on it, question the desire. It's not sexy up front, but the clarity of knowing what you want and having the direction and drive to get it is. Find the real root of what you are after. Get what you need <u>and</u> want in your life. By way of action, guide your man into commitment. Not with sex at first, not with mere talk, but by actions of who you are, what you like to do, and what you enjoy as regular activities. As important as sex is, it's only for a little while. You likely know more than men, that the conversation is the relationship and even if he is good in bed, until his receptors grow in, it's unlikely you will have him in bed for very long before he finds another woman. Stimulate him in other ways first. Just by your presence alone you're enough. The rest of the fun is extra and reserved for the man that earns it through commitment to you.

Final Thoughts | Loving Thoughts

In the beginning of the section, I mentioned that love cannot be intellectualized or thought about. I still stand behind that statement but thinking can keep love alive <u>after</u> it has been experienced. Thoughts of loved ones that are still here or passed still activates dormant neural circuitry and pathways that once were unconscious. Love again resurfaces by looking at a photograph or hearing an old song or smelling a scent that was present during an experience with your beloved or loved ones. Thoughts can strengthen love and the kept image of our loved ones in our mind, as well as felt in our heart, keeps us on the path of a flourishing life.

<u>Closing questions:</u>

How are you performing the small things in your life?

What habits do you want to form?

What can you practice more of?

What's your philosophy of living and loving?

Who are five people you are grateful for and why?

Who could you give unconditional love to today?

CHAPTER 3:

Models: Figures of Excellence

"There is no golden road to excellence;
excellence is the golden road."
— Jim Afremow

What is Excellence? It stems from the Greek word arete meaning moral virtue, high standards of any kind referring to fulfillment of one's purpose or potential to serve in the community. The Greeks mentality of this they called Paideia, meaning to educate and form. Education was delivered by adults within the social group itself, usually nobility that were skilled in arts of war, craftsmanship and the sensual arts. Young men strove to embody qualities such as physical strength and endurance, courage, sense of duty and honor and all virtues suitable for warriors that were lived by their ancestors. Those ancestors were their models.

Niccolò Machiavelli , the Italian political philosopher, understood this concept of models. In his book *The Prince*. He speaks of how a prince should conduct himself and his government by ways of studying history and actions of great men.

"As for the exercise of the mind, a prince must read histories and actions of great men so as to see how they conducted themselves in war and examine the reasons for their victories and defeat in order to imitate the former and avoid the latter. Above all, the prince must follow the example of some great man of the past, who in turn followed the example of another great man who had been praised and honored before him, always keeping his predecessor's deeds and actions in mind."[70]

In today's modern world, things are not much different. The delivery and the way we reach our models may have changed but the influence and desire to emulate our models haven't. In fact, with social media, the internet and improvements in transportation, we can hear about a person of influence from thousands of miles away in seconds and potentially meet them at events or gatherings over night through transportation by way of airplanes and cars.

Even if you're not into sports or movies or any type of celebrities, mathematics, biology, architecture, education, and government all have models as well. They come from all walks of life, sex and creed. What they all have in common though, is a set of traits or values that produce results we could collectively agree is part of a good life.

Seeing the results and success they have, many people want to know how these people acquired their riches, fame, brilliance and beauty. Before I move further, I'd like to say, yes some people do get lucky. They are born into good positions. Some of it is genetic. They have healthy, resilient bodies with particular aptitudes for sport or thinking. What most people neglect to notice is that even with all that, they had to be molded, they found a coach or parent or model or possibly an image or sound that if not directly, indirectly shaped their character, their values and how they conducted themselves in their daily life. Left to figure it out for themselves, they would have unlikely produced anything extraordinary. They didn't do it alone. All the tangible things about these people could be stripped away and they may miss them, that's natural but what's certain is they remain true to a character, a mode of operating that come hell or high water they are committed to a process, dedicated to an ideal, confident in their abilities to come back again and again and win over and over and over until it's done. Until they're done.

I have a list below of some of the people who have influenced me as well as many others. We will learn a little about each and then the traits many of these people possess.

The Models

Greg Plitt[71]

A Baltimore, Maryland Native, Greg Plitt grew up playing football, golf and wrestling in which he was a two time All-American and three time All-State wrestling champion. His inspiration for work outs came when his dad bought a home gym set when he was in the sixth grade then was further pulled toward the military after his sister's transformation after graduating from the United States Naval Academy. Graduating high school in 1996, he then went on to attend the United States Military Academy at West Point graduating in 2000. He was both Airborne and Ranger certified, serving five years as a Ranger.

After his military career, he was seen at a hotel lobby meeting up with friends and asked if he had ever modeled by a photographer. Though he had not, the agent who was asking encouraged him to put together a portfolio and do a shoot with him and being ambitious he did. That was the beginning of his modeling career. He went on to have the most covers of any male model ever, being on a fitness magazine cover every month for five years straight and producing successful programs such as MFT28 on bodybuilding.com and workouts and nutrition guides as well as philosophies on his own site GregPlitt.com. He has starred in films and TV shows like Grudge Match, Terminator, Mystery Millionaire, Watchmen, Workout in the Zone and much more. He was a trainer in LA and an MET-Rx athlete.

Grant Cardone[72,73]

From Lake Charles, Louisiana, Grant Cardone had big dreams of getting rich and building businesses. His model was his dad coming up. His father's work ethic and drive to take care of him, his two brothers, sister and mother was inspiring. His whole life changed though at ten years old when his father died from a heart attack. They had to sell the dream home on the lake his father had bought for the family just months after moving in. He watched his mother close up with fear about how she was going to take care of the family with the death insurance money from his father's passing and what jobs she could take with four kids.

In those early years, he didn't know how to deal with the stress and turned to drugs and alcohol from ages 15 to 25. In that time, he attended Mcneese State University graduating with an economics degree but still continued living poorly. After his mother had had enough of his behavior and getting severely beaten by thugs and getting fired from his first 5 jobs, Grant decided to turn his life around. He entered a rehab program to get clean and once cleaned, he made amends with his mother and borrowed $3000 US dollars from her to enter a sales program that would enable him to increase his skills and income at the car dealership he was currently working in.

From age 25-31 he worked 6 days a week there on top of starting another business that was symbiotic to the first job. He studied real estate and would travel to properties in his free time scoping out the best deals. At age 29 he bought his first single family home, and rented it to two women who for a while paid on time and were good tenants until they one day decided to move and he was now stuck with the payments. Realizing he now had to focus on finding tenants and his other job he sold the house immediately and found a new means to increase income in the same arena.

Still saving almost everything he earned at age 33 he bought his first apartment building in San Diego. It was a 48 unit apartment building in Vista California putting down $350,000. Then a month later he bought 38 units in Point Loma and 3 months after that he bought 92 units. Over a period of 3 years he acquired 500 units and hasn't stopped since. He has built over five businesses that net over $100 million each and owns a real estate portfolio of over 4,000 units worth an excess of $700 million. In his other five successful businesses, Grant Cardone raises millions of dollars for charities and people who have been in natural disasters as well as coach young business people and companies who increase income and help add value to their customers. He has also written several books on how to persuade, close deals and win in our personal lives.

Ed Mylett[74]

As one of the 50 wealthiest Americans under 50 now, Ed Mylett grew up in an average family with dysfunction and substance abuse in Diamond Bar California. Into his teen years he played sports and was always engaged with athletics. He attended the University of the Pacific Stockton earning a bachelor's in communications and played for the NCAA division one Tigers. He went on to be a Three time All American and the NCAA leader in stolen bases.

After graduating and getting an injury that sidelined a promising career in the major leagues, he needed work. Now in his early 20's he moved back into his childhood home for support. His father, noticing a negative attitude forming from the disappointment of not fullinging the dream of playing professional baseball and having attended sobriety meetings for alcoholics, told him that he had a job he could do that would change that. He was at an under-privileged boys center being a counselor and this is when his life began to change.

He dedicated himself to the service of these young men under his care and supervision. Giving them advice and listening to their stories of how they got there and what they wanted for their lives as well as how to overcome the challenges they faced.

Then he got a call from his best friend's dad, who offered him part time work in a financial company. Not very interested in the money side but rather the service end of the business, he poured himself into learning math and business to help people get their money right and their life in order. He eventually became a leader in what is known as World Financial Group and invested in real estate growing his earnings into the hundreds of millions of dollars. He has written the book called #MaxOut and has a podcast and YouTube channel to educate and inspire people to be the best version of themselves.

Arthur Williams[75]

Arthur "Art" Williams grew up in Cairo, Georgia. Sports being a big part of his coming up, he found his passion and love was in football, particularly coaching. He would use his knowledge of coaching and strategy of football to later coach and guide the people he worked with.

His ignition came at age 23 when his father died and the whole life insurance policy his father had left his family underinsured. At age 28, he was introduced to a term life policy by his cousin. With this new information and wanting to help others who were currently in or had experienced what he had when a member of the family dies without the right kind of insurance, he joined his cousin in selling term life at ITT Financial Services. Before this company went out of business he joined Waddell & Reed insurance company, excelling in the field as a salesman earning the title of RVP or Regional Vice President.

Again dissatisfied with the way the corporation was being run, he and 85 other associates formed their own company called A.L Williams & Associates under the motto "Buy Term and Invest the Difference." With his southern hospitality and the sense he was making to the customers, A.L Williams became the largest seller of life insurance in the U.S. They are now known as Primerica Financial Services. In 2008, his net worth was estimated to be $1.4 billion. With this money he has saved sports teams on the verge of going extinct and enriched the community with a spirit of unity and competition. He erased Christian Liberty University of Virginia's debt by donating $70 million dollars to the school. He's written five books and is most well known for his "Just Do It" speech given in 1987 to the National Religious Broadcasters Organization.

The "Colonel" Harland David Sanders[79,80,81,82]

The oldest of three, born in 1890, David Sanders knew and enjoyed work. Being born on an 80-acre farm and seeing his father work and having his mother guide him in disciplines, (no alcohol, no tobacco, no whistling on Sunday; church rule) he learned about responsibility and taking care of himself. Then at six years old, his father died.

Due to lack of funds in the family at the time, his mother had to work several jobs and his was placed in charge of his siblings. His mother had taught him how to cook and bake bread and was skilled in handling meats at age of seven. When his mother wasn't around, he and his siblings would forge fruits and vegetables, herbs and spices to cook for the family that evening. At age 10 he found work as a farmhand.

After his mother remarried, Sanders, now age 13, was not fond of his new stepfather and left town finding work painting horse carriages. At the age of 16 he falsified his age to join the US Army but one year later, his commander, upon finding out his age, had him honorably discharged. He had a couple more unrelated jobs in his teens. One as a railway blacksmith, and a fireman, then decided to study law at La Salle Extension University. He practiced law for three years before getting into a physical fight with his client.

After that he would be in a ferry boat crossing service which became successful. He sold that business and invested the money into selling acetylene lamps for a short time before that venture fell through. Without work again, he moved to Winchester, Kentucky to work as a salesman for Michelin tire which again was a short streak of success before the company closed. Fortunately he met one of the managers and was given the opportunity to run a service station and once more was closed due to the Great Depression.

Shell oil then offered him a job at a service station where he began to serve foods like chicken, ham and steaks. Here is where he began to finalize his "secret recipe" which would later become KFC. Around that time he was commissioned as a Kentucky colonel. His popularity grew. He had acquired a motel that would later burn down and he would rebuild into a 140 seat restaurant. Then as WWII began, gas was being rationed, tourism came to a halt and he was forced to close the station and motel. He then ran cafeterias for the government as an assistant manager.

In 1952 he franchised his secret recipe and began selling Kentucky fried chicken. Having some success in this new store was again short lived so he sold it due to lack of traffic in the town. Now at age 65, he began traveling to find a new place to franchise his chicken. Sometimes sleeping out of his car to meet new people, visit new restaurants, cook his chicken for people and if they liked it negotiate a franchise with them.

At 73 years old he sold the American franchises to two businessmen for $2 million. He held onto the foreign franchises and traveled around the United States visiting other stores, doing quality checks and engaging with its customers and employees. He believed deeply in his service and his product and made it very clear that if it wasn't good he wasn't going to tolerate it. He was known to visit stores and push food onto the floor if it was unsatisfactory.

He died in 1980 at 90 years old. At the time of his death KFC was doing $2 billion in sales annually.

Tony Robbins[83]

As many people may know him as he is now, rich, famous and influential, Tony Robbins grew up poor in North Hollywood with a physically abusive drug and alcohol addicted mother and a dad that wasn't ever around. Being the oldest of two other siblings, he naturally became interested in finding ways to use psychology to calm his mother's episodes down and soothe his brother and sister.

His father was a truck driver, which he never saw much and when he did, they didn't have much to say to one another. His parents, before they were divorced, wanted him to step into the same position his father was in, making $24,000 a year but Tony had a feeling he could do more. At 17, he was a janitor and moved furniture on the weekend for extra money to help his mother and the family. One of the people he helped one day was a family friend who had become educated, earned an above average income and was living well. Tony, being interested in people and how this man achieved his successes, asked about all of it.

This man turned him to someone named Jim Rohn, a self-made millionaire from Idaho farm country who was giving self development seminars. A seminar ticket was $35 and Tony was only making $40 a week. He took the risk, made the investment in himself and bought the ticket. After hearing about the seminar, Tony approached Jim Rohn. After a brief interaction, Tony asked if he could come work and shadow him. Mr. Rohn hired him and from there he learned more about behavioral psychology, developed his self development seminars, wrote his first book and became a millionaire by age twenty-six. He's now worth over $400 million at age 58. One of the most valuable things he believes helped him help millions of people and still does today because of the advice Jim Rohn gave him. It is simply to "work harder on yourself than you do your job. If you work hard on your job, you can make a living. If you work hard on yourself, you can make a fortune."

Jim Rohn[84,85]

Jim came from a loving family in Idaho. His mother was French and his father was German. Each bi-lingual and hard working. His father owned a farm with livestock and growing up Jim would wake early to tend to the cows and other animals. His first job was milking cows. From working that job he developed a way of thinking that later he would incorporate into his life philosophies. Up until age 25 he lived a mediocre life. He did one year of college, dropped out and started working for the department store called Sears. He got married and started a family and had found himself lacking in his finances, his relationships and falling short of his promises.

It all changed one day a Girl Scout came to the door selling Girl Scout cookies. She had a wonderful sales pitch and was very confident and then asked for the order. Jim didn't have any money though so he did the next best thing and told her a lie that he had already bought some cookies from another Girl Scout. With kindness the little girl thanked him for his time and left. Once this little girl left and he closed the door, he felt a deep remorse for lying to a child and terrible for being broke. He swore to himself he never wanted to feel like that again.

One day at work a friend was telling him about a successful businessman who would give seminars on self development and self growth named John Earl Shoaff. Earl Shoaff was an entrepreneur who started a direct selling company called Abundavita. In 1955, Jim Rohn joined this business with him and then in 1957, resigned from Abundavita and joined Nutra-Bio with Earl Shoaff and for the next five years Earl mentored Jim. Using the lessons he had learned from his new mentor, Jim Rohn built one of the largest organizations in the company and expanded into Canada. With this great success he was promoted to vice president of Nutra-Bio. This company went out of business in the 1960s but by then Jim had become successful financially, well educated and developed as a leader. He was invited to talk at Earl Shoaff's Rotary club. In 1963 he gave his first seminar at the Beverly Hills hotel. His seminars would grow to include thousands of people and dozens of countries around the world. He did this for over 40 years before he died in 2009. He inspired people like Mark R. Hughes, founder of HerbalLife International and Performance Coach and motivational speaker Tony Robbins.

John "Jocko" Willink[86]

Once a young rebellious kid from New England, who rocked out to black flag and embraced a hardcore discipline mindset, John "Jocko" Willink went on to become an elite member of the US Navy, earning the rank of Commander. In starting his 20 year career in the SEAL teams, he learned some hard lessons about listening, humility and sacrifice. He has a podcast called Jocko's Podcast where he and his now training and business partner discuss leadership, ownership, humility, training principles and cover military history, strategy and how it applies to business and relationships in the civilian world. He's the founder of Echelon Front, co-founder of Origin USA and Jocko Supplements.

Marcus Luttrell[87,88,89,90]

Made well known after Operation Red Wings, Marcus Luttrell was the only man alive after being attacked by Taliban in Kunar Province, a mountainous terrain with limited places to get cover. One hour into the attack, his team mate Danny Dietz was wounded. In an attempt to get them out of there, Marcus picked him up to jump down to a safe position, but in doing so, spun his teammate into a bullet by accident, killing him instantly. Unprepared for the weight of his teammate falling over top of him, it collapsed him, flipping him off the rock embankment in which he face planted into a boulder breaking his nose, biting his tongue off and swallowing it. Now on all fours, he regurgitates it and holds it in his mouth. His other teammate, Mike Murphy went to a precipice to get a satellite phone signal to call for reinforcements and was shot dead.

As Marcus seeks cover again, he links up with his teammate Matthew Axelrod for a moment before an RPG (rocket propelled grenade) blast separated them. Axelrod was never seen again. Murphy's call signaled eight members of the 160th Special Operations Aviation Regiment and eight more Navy SEALS into action. As the aircraft flew over the mountains and the team prepared to rope down, a 12-year old boy serving as an insurgent fired an RPG that struck the fuel tanks killing everyone aboard.

Marcus was knocked unconscious and when he awoke, he was laying on a rock with only his upper body gear on, one magazine of 30 rounds and a harness. He was paralyzed from the waist down. He crawled to cover nearby as the sun began to set. He then reached out and grabbed a rock and drew a line in the dirt in front of him and crawled through it until his feet hit and if he was still alive, he told himself, he would do it again.

He did this for 7 miles until he found a ravine to drink from and while there was found by a man named Mohammad Gulab and other villagers. Gulab and the villagers protected Luttrell from the Taliban, considering it their duty under what they call "Pashtunwali" a tribal honor code. Not long after arriving in the village, a team of Army Rangers landed and picked up Luttrell. These two men have remained friends ever since.

> "It takes more than one voice to help us to see, to help us to think, to help us to make decisions, to help us to evaluate, it takes a variety of personalities, messages, points of view. The weight of experience, if it comes from several sources, can be of incredible value when you sum-total it."
> —Jim Rohn

Virtues of High Achieving People

• **Belief**

What kind of belief? Self Belief. Not in who you are but what you are. Not your title, your name, or any external thing but what you are inwardly.

• **Commitment**

Telling yourself you don't care how hard something is or how long it takes- you will do whatever it takes morally and ethically to get the results. Then actually do what you said you would do, long after the mood you said it in has passed. A prime example of this is Mozart. In pursuing mastery, he played piano so frequently his hands became deformed. Grant Cardone is another example. After meeting his now

Wife, Elena, he called twice a week for thirteen months asking her out after being flat out told "No, I'm not interested" almost every time.

They know the results they want and they see it as the present and commit to making it reality.

• Confidence

Where does confidence come from? Overcoming consistent, difficult circumstances. How does that help? You know you can control your response to any circumstance that arises. It's a must to maintain the character traits of excellence no matter what happens. It's being secure that your best effort is enough even when you don't win; That you are doing things right and seeking continual progress. It's living up to your standard of success.

Ask yourself:

Am I meeting my own standard Excellence?

If you are not, change it.

If you are, good. Keep doing that.

> "Success does not define us, we define the success."
> — Greg Plitt

Urban Meyer's, University of Cincinnati Football coach has what he calls the "success equation". It looks like this:

$$E + R = O$$

Events + Response = Outcome

Events are going to happen every day. Right now, even with nothing going on around you, it's an event in your life. It may be small or quiet but it's happening. You don't control that part. How you respond to the event, what's happening around you is yours to control and that will determine the outcome of the event. Particularly in loss, in failure, with mistakes, you are better able to determine the outcome by your response. You can lose and still be a winner by having a winning spirit and keeping your cool. With that attitude, another opportunity will arise to win.

• Cool Under Pressure

When high stress situations arise, say in a tournament with seconds on the clock to win, or getting struck by a tough opponent, or a disgruntled customer begins getting emotional, the successful professionals are calm, confident and in control of their bodies and emotions. They can maintain a level head and operate efficiently and swiftly to provide solutions. Even when adrenaline is high and their hearts are pounding, they use it as a way to focus and gain the upper hand on the situation. They obtain this ability by hours and hours of training, practice and study.

• Consistent

These people didn't just do something once or twice or even three times. They regularly show up and keep showing up until they get to where they need to be. Everyday they are training in some way. Every day they are working in some aspect of their vision and ideal self and outcomes. It's mostly small things. They don't run marathons everyday, or raise millions of dollars every hour or finish entire projects in one swing. They bite off what they can chew and go from there. That keeps them in the game and able to manage the environment around them. What they cannot manage, they delegate to someone who's stronger in that area.

• Coachable

They can be taught and implement advice well. That sounds simple and easy but many people are not very coachable. They may hear but don't listen or they can watch but cannot imitate. Michael Jordan was renowned for his coachability and it led him to be able to sharpen his skill set above his competitors. These types of people are, in a word, humble. They know there is more to learn and are willing to surrender what they know as their way for a way that's possibly better.

• **Discipline**

> Discipline equals Freedom."
> —Jocko Willink

Successful people in all endeavors don't waiver in their commitments, drive or process. They do what they are supposed to do, when they're supposed to do it, especially when they don't feel like it or don't want to. They do this with the knowledge they will be able to do what they want to do when they want to do it when they have created the habits and patterns to effortlessly perform.

Do they fail?
All the time.

Do they have days where things don't go right?
Of course.

Do they still have desires and urges?
Yes.

The difference is, they don't act on them as they arise. They are aware of them and see if they are compatible with the end result they need. If those desires are not, they stay away from that person, place or thing that will hinder progress until it won't.

They hold the line. They work on it until it works. That doesn't mean always in the same way but they find a way.

• Dedication

They have a single minded loyalty towards a person or activity. They devote quality time, and energy towards developing their skills in their career, their bodies, mind and relationships. When obstacles arise they maintain focus on the task in front of them. They know where they are going and will stay on the path until they get to where they need to be.

• Delayed Gratification

The people who win the most, who achieve financial freedom, who have strong loving relationships with friends and spouses and are the happiest with themselves all delay gratification in the moment for future gain.

> "Pay the price today so you can
> pay any price tomorrow."
> —Grant Cardone

> "We always invest today, sacrifice
> today for tomorrow's betterment."
> —Greg Plitt

"My vitamin is the future. I live on a future."
—Grant Cardone

They acknowledge the desire they have now and then visualize the outcome they want. If the thing they want now and the thing they need in the future don't align, they subordinate the feeling and do the thing they know will lead to or has led to consistent desired results even though they don't feel like it or don't want to do it. They embrace short term pain for long term gain.

• **Embrace the Suck**

A term military personnel use during training and other wretched experiences that in essence means things are the way they are, bitching about it, complaining and gripping won't make the situation better. Embracing adversity and using it has the opportunity to find a silver lining and use the pain as fuel. The next time you think something sucks, just remember, the suck is your old self dying and a new you being forged.

• **Foresight**

"Vision without action is a dream.
Action without vision is a nightmare."
— Japanese Proverb

Most people see but have no vision. They can see what's in front of them but not the big picture. The most successful among us at work, in sports, in business and on the battlefield have the quality of foresightedness; the ability to see what happens before it happens.

This type of vision widens our perspective and determines the overall context of events, not just what is happening at the moment. The idea is to think about the consequences of the actions we take and what could and needs to happen long term for mission success.

How does one develop foresightedness?

Training in that arena. Consistent and persistent study across related and unrelated fields, connecting the things that may seem unrelated. 3M is a master at this. In 3M, they have many talented and educated people across domains that will at times create things that had promise in the idea stage but fall flat once produced. They don't just throw it out though. They record it, leave it aside or push it into other departments to see where it could be used. Others are free to try to use it in other areas. This how Post-it notes came about.

In 1968 Dr. Spence Silver, a 3M scientist, was experimenting one day looking to make a super strong adhesive. Instead he made a very weak one that could be removed without residue. After 3 years of looking for a use for this new adhesive, a colleague, Art Fry was attending a seminar by Dr. Silver and the idea struck him when he heard about the adhesive: it would hold his page in the books he was reading whereas his other book markers would just fall out. In 1980, they became known nationwide.

Another way to be foresighted is asking questions. Going through theoretical scenarios and thinking of the multiple possibilities. Questions like:

If I do this, what could possibly happen?

See at least three possibilities. See the best outcome, the worst outcome and what to do if nothing happens. Think about the problem working itself out over time. Think about the possible unforeseen problems that could loom larger than what is currently happening at this moment. With this style of contingency planning, you will cover all bases.

> "If only it were possible for us to see farther
> than our knowledge reaches, and yet a little way
> beyond the outworks of our divining, perhaps we
> would endure our sadnesses with greater confi-
> dence than our joys."[92]
> —Rainer Maria Rilke

Foresightedness also requires a detachment from the present moment. A view from above like being on a balcony. While on a balcony, you can see obstacles hundreds of feet before the person below even becomes aware of something in their path. As a leader, you can now communicate to the people in the field about what's coming up and then collaborate on how to overcome, get through or go around the obstacles to get to the next checkpoint or final result.

Prince Philopoemen of Achaeans, General of the Achaean League is an example of foresightedness.[92] In people who studied him, they found that even in times of peace he was thinking of ways to wage war.

Once when riding in the hills of his country with friends, he stopped and asked them: "If the enemy were up in those hills and we were here with our army, who would have the advantage? How could we attack without breaking formation? If we wanted to retreat, how would we do that? If they were to retreat, how would we pursue them?"

This created a conversation between the men and as his friends explained their opinions, he would listen carefully then give his detailed explanation in response. This type of visualizing kept his mind sharp and ready for adversity as well as for victory. This same General was the one who led a victory over the Spartans in 207 CE.

Alexander The Great was said to regularly hunt when he was not at war. Hunting kept his mind and body fit for battle. He would be able to use animals rather than people to try strategies and maneuvers on as well as practice using his weapons.

• **Fear**

Yes. Elite performers all feel it. In fact, they likely know it better than the average person. The difference is two-fold.

1) They channel it
2) They think of it in a useful way

By channeling I mean they focus that energy, the adrenaline into performing. It makes their focus razor sharp and brings them into the present moment.

When they feel the rush before a race, speaking to a crowd or just danger in general, they know it's their body priming them to perform. They're excited about the rush and know it's to help them. Some call it "racehorse nerves" meaning our body is gearing up to be at peak readiness to give us the best performance. It's the same rush that stops many people, makes them shake with nervous energy. It isn't to inhibit or stifle performance. It's our mighty horsepower and it's to be reined in and guided to give our best on stage or in the arena.

• **Finisher**

They finish what they are doing. They see it through to the end. Other people may organize and may persuade them into something that has been started but they will finish what is theirs and what they commit to. They may have many projects open but the central priority project is focused on until completion. They don't work to simply work. They work for a particular result and the only way that happens is finishing.

• **Grit**

> "A man can only be defeated in two
> ways: if he gives up or he dies."[95]
> —Richard Machowicz

When things get tough, when things get hard, successful people get tougher, they go harder or they enter what Marcus Luttrell has called "the low gear" and grind it out until the mission is complete. Nothing will stop them but themselves or death. Marcus Luttrell is an example of grit.

• **Growth Mindedness**

This term was popularized by Carol Dweck. She defines two kinds of mindsets.

1) Fixed Mindset
2) Growth Mindset

A fixed mindset is when someone believes their basic qualities, like their intelligence or talent, are fixed traits. They think they were born that way and they will remain that way.

A growth mindset is when someone believes that their most basic abilities can be developed through dedication and hard work. No matter where they are they believe they can become better through hard work, study and practice.

Dweck performed a study based on these two mindsets to see if students could learn more by encouraging them to work harder and practice rather than just testing for IQ. In Dweck's paper, "Implicit Theories of Intelligence Predict Achievement Across Adolescent Transition" she studied high school students in New York and found that their theories of intelligence affected their math grades. Over a period of two years, those with a fixed mindset declined in academic performance while those with a growth mindset excelled.

Dweck then designed an eight week program that would teach the below average students study skills and how they could become more intelligent. Another group, the control group, was taught the study skills but not Dweck's theory of intelligence. After two months the students in the growth mindset group that were previously falling behind were now improving substantially whereas the control group was not.

In short, the best always praise people for their efforts, not their talents and only reward for results, which in a sense they earned themselves by doing the work and learning the skills.

• Ownership

They feel a deep need to take responsibility for the results produced by their own doing, their teams, and their organizations. They accept faults and failure as their own even when they personally did not commit them. No, that doesn't mean they take blame for the sake of taking blame or because they are trying to save anyone. It means they believe if they were in proximity, they could have influenced the situation and changed the situation for the better. Then with candor and tact, they collaborate on how they can improve the next time so as to avoid the same mistake.

An excellent example of this was in 2006 in the city of Ramadi, Iraq where the epicenter of the insurgency was located during the war. At this time, Jocko Willink was in charge of operations conducted by US Navy SEALS.[96] Multiple other elements were in coordination with this band of men including allied Iraqi soldiers. During this particular operation, mistakes were made through lack of communication between the men combined with poor judgement. A firefight ensued. Only it wasn't with the enemy, it was at the time, unknowingly with themselves; fratricide or a blue on blue. Once the firefight stopped, one friendly Iraqi soldier was dead, two more including a SEAL were wounded and the rest of the men were shaken up.

This was sent up the chain of command. Being that Jocko was the commanding officer in charge of that SEAL element, he would be giving a debrief to the leaders in charge of him as well as the AAR (after action review) with his men. He was going over and detailing who took the shots, who communicated the okay to fire and who caused the death of the Iraqi soldier and wounded men. While doing this he had the option of assigning blame, pointing the finger or taking ownership. He knew who was in charge of the operation, he knew who was responsible to make sure communications were clear and plans were understood. With that knowledge he walked into the room with his commanding officer, master chief, and investigating officer waiting with the rest of his team. He asked a simple question:

Who's fault is this?

As each man on the team took a turn to speak and take responsibility for the failed mission, Jocko turned it down. Then he explained, knowing he may well lose his job and possibly credibility with his men, that he was to blame. He was the commanding officer in charge of the operation, in charge of making sure the plan was understood and that his men were safe. Then he went over what they could do to avoid this from happening again. He knew that to maintain his integrity as a leader and a man, he had to take ownership no matter the cost to him.

Instead of being fired and losing credibility, the opposite happened. They respected and trusted him more. The other members of the team were inspired and cohesion between the team strengthened. In short, the more a team takes responsibility and ownership of its problems, the more those problems will get solved.

• Passion

Some people call it "heart power". Some call it the "fire inside". Most know it as passion: an intense enthusiasm for an activity or people in our lives. People who win consistently have a borderline obsession with their craft, for their company and for their people. It's the fuel that drives them when the chips are down and it's how they excel, master the basics and greater levels of complexity and challenge. It's a deep love for what they do and it's a requirement for being successful in anything. Those without passion and still obtain what others call "success", is a personal failure. Those that don't have passion for something, don't go as far as those that do.

• Persistence

A challenge is to elevate you, it's a chance to use your skills and knowledge, to see how much you really want this circumstance, this particular outcome. An analogy of persistence is that of a plant coming through concrete. It pushes and grows and finds a way through to the surface because it wants to live, it wants to survive. It doesn't care how difficult the task is. It keeps pushing and trying until it makes it through or until it dies.

As people, instead of focusing on how hard our task is, we are better served when we focus on our drive and system to overcome or get through our task just like flowers that find a way or make a way through a hard surface. When you come through, you will create value. Internally for you so self-worth and externally for others in the form of wisdom, greater potential, becoming a leader, a teacher, a coach.

• **Pivot**

When plans fail as they inevitably do at times, these people take the same drive and energy that was focused on one goal and turn it to the next one. They never quit. They may stop one thing or change the approach to the endeavor but they keep their essence, their spirit intact and bring it to where they are going.

Do they mourn for a period?

Yes. Not very long though.

How long? Depends on the loss or disappointment but I would say no longer than a week for minor issues. Something major could take years but they find a way to move through it. Remember, yes. Reflect. Dwell, no. They don't live there, they acknowledge what happened, unpack it, then put it aside and move forward.

• **Positivity**

Their attitude towards life is that the glass is half full. They find the silver lining and are able to use it to get through negative situations and learn.

Science has found the brain works up to 31% better in a positive frame of mind. This means that when grappling on the mats, lifting, or negotiating, staying positive, seeing the good, believing things can work in your favor, puts you at an advantage.

• **Presentness**

Being in the moment. The only way we can rectify the past or influence the future is by taking action in the present moment. It's okay to reflect dispassionately, to gather information from the past to use now and for upcoming events but to dwell is detrimental to growth. "You don't live there anymore" is a reminder of being here now, the past is for experience and the future is for inspiration. They pull from each in the moment to excel forward.

• **Preparation**

They prepare every day for high-pressure moments through training, practice and ongoing efforts in their craft.

When someone fails to prepare it means they are preparing to fail. Being prepared for the day, having something as small as your work clothes out and ready, your breakfast pre-made and in the fridge, bags packed and set out to go, makes the next step of taking action seamless. In fact, you may look forward to taking action or doing more because you know how fluid you can be now, it's attractive. In the big picture of life, having a plan of what to do when failure happens or tragedy strikes, what to do next when your plan succeeds, where you want to be in the next one to ten years and having the next step ready and known, makes staying on the path easy when distraction, appetites and passions try to lure you in and they will try to, so be aware.

Plans change, circumstances change but that's why we make them. We have something we can adapt and mold to instead of being blinded by fear or joy. We have a map and compass of how to maneuver over the territory.

• Resilience

The ability to move through hardship and become better by it. Mentally, physically, and emotionally, all negatively that impacts them is used as a vehicle to get where they want to be and become who they want to be. Again they read, research, study, train hard, practice and surround themselves with the images and people who are doing well despite obstacles and setbacks. They draw upon these images and knowledge in the moment and when it gets tough, they find a way to keep moving toward their ideal.

• Self-Control

> "One can have no smaller or greater
> mastery than mastery of oneself."
> —Leonardo Da Vinci

High performers can identify the things they can control and ignore everything else. Like all of us, they still feel, they still have deep emotions and desires. The difference is they don't act on them until it's appropriate or useful.

The theologian Reinhold Niebuhr summed it up well when he said:

God, grant me the serenity to accept the things I cannot change, the courage to change the things I can, and the wisdom to know the difference.

Even if you are not religious the statement contains a truth. We do not control our external environment. Yes, we have thermostats and you may be a team leader who makes the plans or head of the household but life doesn't care about that. Those things still aren't yours. Plans fail, items break and titles can be taken away. What we have the most control over is how we think, how honest we are and how we respond. They are the keys to influencing the outside world and how it affects our life, as well as those around us.

• **Sacrifice**

There is no such thing as success without giving something of value in return for what you receive. Be it time, energy, money, relationships, or a combination of these. It comes at a price.

> "There is no such thing as climbing
> to the top obstacle free."
> —John C. Maxwell

Everything worth having in life has a price on it. It's not always going to be monetary either, though it may entail spending to earn the skills, the experience and the knowledge. As we are wired, we have sacrifice to:

1) Appreciate and value the wins
2) Understand loss and learn

• **Humility**

One of the best ways I've heard humility spoken of is by Author Eric Greitens, former Navy Seal who starts and ends his day with this mantra:

I begin with humility, I act with humility, I end with humility. Humility leads to an open mind and a forgiving heart. With an open mind and a forgiving heart, I see every person as superior to me in some way; with everyone as my teacher, I grow in wisdom. As I grow in wisdom, humility becomes ever more my guide. I begin with humility, I act with humility, I end with humility.

Humility is the ability to subordinate yourself to the mission or goal, meaning the mission or goal and the people involved come before you. Your mindset is that of service. Does that mean neglect your needs? No. Does it mean your needs may lie fallow for a moment? Yes. If everyone works together with humility though, you will be taken care of.

Many of you may have heard the story of the over-flowing teacup. The student and the master have been training for a while. The student is arrogant and believes that he knows enough and that his master's simple exercises are not that helpful any longer. In a sense he's a "know it all". One day they were having tea and the master asked the student if he would like some. The student responded "yes" and the master proceeded to pour tea into his cup. As the cup began to fill up, he continued to pour even though the cup was overflowing. Bewildered, the student says to the master who seemed unaware: "the cup is full, it cannot be filled anymore, why are you still pouring?"

The master responded "You are like this tea cup, so full that nothing more can be added. Come back when the cup is empty. Come back with an empty mind. Only then can something be added."

If we are to grow more, we must listen and be available to try something new, to see it another way. Keeping our experience available as well but being able to set that down so long as the risk is low and see if another way is better.

• Hunger

Successful people want more. More what? More of what makes them enjoy life. It's what Ed Mylett calls "blissfully dissatisfied." For example, for those who eat steak, let's say you get the all-time quality cut. It's seared and grilled to perfection. You take your first bite and swallow. It's delightful. You aren't satisfied though are you? And when you're done with the entire steak you may be satiated for the next few hours but if someone offered you that meal again you would likely do it again wouldn't you?

Hunger in any arena is the same way. The successful professionals are pulled into their work again and again hungry for the next win, hungry for the next lesson, the next discovery, the next session or insight. They are never satisfied with just one time. They crave the experience and the result over and over.

• Tenacity

Persistent determination.

This is Derek Clark's favorite word.
Derek Clark is a six time best selling author and a talented rapper. He was given up for adoption as a young boy and

was in several different foster homes over the period of 13 years. He had what psychologists labeled "erratic psychosis" and didn't learn to read until 9 years old. Then one day he met somebody that believed in him and helped reveal his gifts and develop his ability. By the time he was 25, he made his first $100,000 by the time he was 31, he made his first million.

Many others including motivational speaker Les Brown have been through similar situations. A common virtue among all successful people is they are doggedly determined to get where they want to be no matter where they currently are. They are, in a word, tenacious.

• Time-Perspective

Similar to foresightedness, time perspective means how much time one spends looking towards the future, where they are presently and pull lessons from the past. Successful people think long-term. They're in what they do for the long-haul. Their jobs, their position they hold or their geographical location may change but their overall mission is based on longevity. They know that **if it is not sustainable it is not successful**, meaning if they cannot have this over the course of their life, they don't invest much or anything into the activity.

They, with great accuracy, can assess how long something can and should take and are willing to make the sacrifice of time if it gets them what they truly want.

The Dichotomy of Excellence

It's been said that most people don't know how good you have to be to just suck in a professional arena. The practice squad for an NFL football team is still better than a majority of college teams. The guy who is the 5th best pitcher in the MLB, is still better than the best guy in the minor leagues. The 3rd place finisher in the olympics could still beat almost anyone who challenges them on the planet in their domain. This doesn't mean they are flourishing or excellent in other areas of their lives, which is a mistake many make when looking up to or involved with high performers.

Someone can be an excellent parent or an excellent friend but in the marketplace, in the competition arena they could only be a tenth place finisher. That doesn't disclaim them from being an excellent performer though. If that's all they could do, if that was their best, they can still execute and perform with excellence and not win.

In contrast, the person in 1st place could be an excellent performer but fail in being excellent in other areas just as important or more important than winning the race or competition. It's only one area and that one area doesn't constitute a good life. Excellence isn't a one time thing either. You don't win once and obtain excellence forever. Excellence is fleeting. Ben Bergeron calls it "chasing excellence". It will always be a pursuit and in pursuing excellence, we are in its draft. In being in its draft, we achieve higher.

I believe there are two types of Excellence:

- Professional Excellence
- Personal Excellence

Though both are related, they are different.

Professional Excellence is specific. It's trained for a particular skill in sport, an art, a trade, a craft.

Personal Excellence is how you live day to day, how you treat yourself, how you treat others, your character.

You can have NBA level skills, have a PhD or be an elite in your field but if you are not humble, if you don't have consistent persistence or resilience, very few people will stay to support you when you are in need. And at the highest level, it's about the people. At first they may support you and mistake arrogance for strength and confidence but as reality unfolds and problems arise they look for true strength of character. Having only talent or having only skill will make you valuable to the business, to the market which is great. We need competent people. It won't make you all you could be to the people though. It's excellence but people need more than just your skills at work. They need you to be excellent in the other areas of life after you are done working.

Personal excellence practiced properly can lead to professional excellence but it has to be a focus of that individual and even then it's very competitive. Nonetheless, the ultimate goal isn't to win the title or all the money or whatever it is you want, that's a consequence. A consequence of becoming the best version of you. The resources and titles and things you need for you and your tribe will come. It starts with you and how you carry yourself in everything you do.

Again, competency is only valuable insofar as you can help other people with it. That could be entertaining them, which most people would rather be entertained than taught or even coached. It could be coaching them though, or making them feel good, teaching them skills but basically getting them the results they want. If you can do that, they will love you. If you only possess one level of excellence though and the palate of the spectators and audience changes, as it always does, then if you have only one level of excellence, you lose.

We see it all the time in sports. An extraordinary athlete wins and wins, makes appearances and shakes hands, has rallies in other arenas. Then they lie or cheat or steal. They have an affair. We as people can understand. We are human. We all have desires. It's the fact that we thought, because they are excellent in one field, disciplined in one area, that they were excellent everywhere and they weren't.

We instinctively trust people of great influence or skill and when they abuse that power or squander it, it can be devastating. Compound the effect with them not taking ownership and we drop them. We can forgive a bad play, a bad season, even a poor attitude for a time on the field or in the marketplace. We don't forget and have a difficult time forgiving an infidelity, a lack of character, a lack of ownership for results.

Remember our models are no different than us in the sense that they're human. Said another way "kill your idols", remove the veil of the illusory projection. They aren't who you think they are. They are who they are and the more you can see them for that, the better you will be able to understand them and yourself.

> "Character supersedes talent
> everyday of the week."
> —Inky Johnson

Personal excellence is something we all can obtain even if our skills and our talents are unremarkable. By working on our skills they can improve radically and in doing so we can build our character better than before and possibly develop into the level of a professional. When we live our day to day, from doing the dishes, cleaning the yard, or listening to a friend, we can practice the virtues of excellence and live a good life.

Mature Performance

In Ander Ericsson's study of deliberate practice, he discusses the differences between adolescent performance and adult performance in relation to music. He says,

"In the performance of music, children and adolescents are judged principally on their technical proficiency. Expert adult performers, however, are judged on their interpretation and ability to express emotions through music.

He then goes on to talk about mathematics.

"Similar considerations may explain why mathematical prodigies can fail as adult mathematicians. The lack of overlap in the performance of precocious children and adult scientists in mathematics is even clearer than in music: Superior ability in mental addition and multiplication demonstrate efficiency in the mechanics of mathematics, whereas major adult contributions in mathematica reflect insights into the structure of mathematical problems and domains. The criteria for eminent performance goes beyond expert mastery of available knowledge and skills and requires an important and innovative contribution to the domain."

In short, it's not just about what you can do, it's what you can do for others, the community. What contribution can you make through your work, through your skills and character?

Finding a Model

> "The only time you should try to measure up to
> someone's idea of who you are or what you're
> capable of is when that person is a role model
> cheering you on."[103]
> —Brendon Burchard

What is a model? And what do they provide us with? A model is a person or idea we admire and emulate. We mirror them because of what they do, how they speak, and the results they produce in their life are what we would like to reproduce in our own lives. They are a source of inspiration when we hit rock bottom, when Murphy's Law is beating us down. They transfer energy to us to take that one more step forward toward who we are striving to become.

Everyone's model of success looks different. There's no one model for everything. Someone can have many models in their life. One for work ethic, one for love, one for finances, one for health. Some may come with it all but it's unlikely and that's okay. Kids usually find this process effortless but as adults it can seem childish or immature. It's not and it's one of the best ways to learn, being that it can reduce the time it takes to find solutions and improve our circumstances.

So what does someone look for in a model and where do we find them and how do we know if they are fit for us?

For me it's the traits above. For you it may differ. I encourage you to make a list of traits and ways of being you find attractive and empowering. Then read that list 3 times a day. Morning, noon and night for 8 weeks. It will keep you aware of people who have them and also remind you of who you'd like to become. The #1 thing common among all great models in any field is they have overcome struggles in their lives. What some would call a "worthy struggle."

What's a worthy struggle?

A worthy struggle is the act of overcoming challenges or obstacles for something greater than yourself and benefits a group of people.

Common examples of this are soldiers fighting for freedom, the single mother or father working three jobs to provide for their family, a poor immigrant coming to America with no money, sleeping in their car, learning the language and educating themselves to improve communications and business between nations.

The struggle is what makes them great. Things that are easy, things that come naturally are taken for granted and don't stimulate consistent action. Hardship, pain, fear, the unknown, possibility, stimulate action. They stimulate the desire to change. I'm not saying create unnecessary problems but I'm saying **your greatness will come from overcoming the struggles in your life.** In your struggle, your fight against weakness, ignorance, and degradation, you will find your potential, then actually become your own ideal image. There is no victory without obstacles, competition, or struggle, even if you are only competing with yourself.

"You are your only competition."
—Anonymous

We don't always have access to the people we'd like to model either because they are from a different era and have died, live far away or are high profile. One way to be in touch with them is to go to the bookstore and look in the sections that contain the information you're looking for then look up the author. YouTube them. Google them. Then if possible go and meet them at a seminar.

If you don't know who would be a good model for you now, ask questions such as:

- If I were living the way I believe to be successful, where would I spend my free time?

- How would they treat others?

- How would they eat?

- How would they walk?

- How would they talk?

- How would a successful person handle adversity?

- How would they handle victory and defeat?

- Who's been where I am in history and overcome their circumstances?

- What would they do if they were here?

Questions like this will allow you to see in yourself the same potential that countless others have realized in the past. By making yourself into the person that is capable of performing the job, building the relationships and closing the deals, **results will come over time.**

Another way to know when a model is fit for you is when you feel communion with them. Communion meaning you begin consciously modeling their traits and incorporating them into your life. Again, the first place that everyone can start to find their models, and I highly recommend, is with books.

A book is good company. It comes to your longing
but pursues you never...it silently serves the soul
without recompense, not even for the hire of love.
And yet more noble, it seems to pass from itself,
and enter the memory, and to hover in silvery
transformation there, until the outward book is
but a body and its soul and spirit are flown to you

and possess your memory like a spirit.
—H. W. Beecher

Now with the internet, we can use search engines and social media but a book is tangible and books contain crystallized thought. It's the distillation of this person's life, ideas, and how they have done the thing you desire to be doing and it's in the palm of your hands. No backlight keeping you up, no batteries needed. Just your energy and the will to focus on the text. It will stimulate your imagination too.

The Good in the Bad

"If only there were evil people somewhere insidiously committing evil deeds, and it were necessary only to separate them from the rest of us and destroy them. But the line dividing good and evil cuts through the heart of every human being. And who is willing to destroy a piece of his own heart?"
—Aleksandr Solzhenitsyn

We don't just learn from the virtuous people in our lives and history. We learn from everyone. People in history, tyrants, criminals, and bad leaders all serve us in a way that allows us to know what not to do, what we don't want and how we may avoid those characters and circumstances from arising in the future. Depending on the endeavor, we may need their machiavellian tactics or their system of organization or their ways of influencing to do good. Like a sieve that filters dirt from water, we must learn to filter the good from the bad in everything. Negative is normal. Negation is part of the success equation and when something comes in the form of the negative, there's a silver lining. There is some good in everything. Find it and use it.

To Model or Not to Model?

> You cannot be what you do not see.
> —Jay Shetty

You may be wondering, "how long should I model someone?"

Answer: Until it no longer serves your purpose or way of being. Until you stop getting the results you want.

Just like with identity when we "try on" our models or mentors shoes, we begin to construct ideas and create feelings of what that life may be like. Kids do this growing up. For example, a little girl pushing a stroller pretending to be a mother, a young boy playing a soldier pretending to be at war. Though this isn't reality, the inspiration sparks action into a field of interest in which we can now practice and begin mapping a pattern of being. Then as we become that persona, we can become a model, a mentor for those around us, young and old.

As we grow up our interests naturally change and evolve as do our bodies, minds and abilities. We are always changing whether we consciously know it or not. We are dynamic. Our bodies totally replace our skeleton structure approximately every 7 years in a process called "remodeling," our lungs cells replace themselves every 8 days and 100 millions new blood cells are being made every minute. Our basic character, our personality and our way of being is difficult to change and usually lasts our life time unless affected by a traumatic event but it's possible for that to change as well.

People desire new things and make sacrifices, doing the work to become more than what they were. Their work changes, their ambitions change and their relationships keep growing and some die off. It will more often than not, be very clear when it's time to move on to the next model or strike off on your own path.

Signs of this are:

- Your priorities or values have changed likely due to age and experience.

- You have a deep understanding of the topic of interest and can predict accurately your models moves.

- You can teach what your model has taught you equally or better than they can.

Model and Modify

Stay with the person you're pulled towards so long as they are moral and ethical in their ways, learn as much as you possibly can from them. If they are not, extract only the good. Much is said in their non-verbal cues, sometimes even more so than in their spoken language. Absorb and then add your own style to it. Then try something new. See if you can then do it better and help more people.

The point of the model isn't to become them. Bruce Lee said it well when he said "Always be yourself, express yourself, have faith in yourself, do not go out and look for a successful personality and duplicate it." The point is to use what serves you in their way of living to become the best version of you. Once you become skilled from shadowing, from being mentored, accept where you are. This allows you to become a light unto yourself. You find that you are capable of more and that you have something to offer that they may not have. We all are unique. We will only pass this way, in this form, one time. Even if we were cloned, our copy wouldn't have the same experiences.

The goal is to see the outside world as it is. See those who are doing well and gather the essence of those people, their character traits and values, then bring that into your own life, living into those values to find out what it's like for you to live that way. You make it your own. Anything that is false will be a misery for you over time because it doesn't align with where you are, with who you are.

Only truth will bring you peace, only truth will bring you happiness, only truth will bring you excellence. Maybe not upfront but truth is the only way we grow better.

There is no escaping you. We cannot attach our goals to people and expect to have a fulfilling life. Using them as a model, as a more efficient and effective way is okay but again it's not where we stay. We must convert what we learn into our own lived experience and into our own circumstances and life's purpose.

When we have a firm understanding of why and how people achieve excellence and then help others to do the same in their lives, we then have gathered the essence of their success. Then we can take it anywhere in our lives. The greatest among us are always themselves. They learned well from successful people, yes but they use what they learned in their own way to create their own style and express themselves.

"Absorb what is useful, discard what is useless and
add what is specifically your own."
—Bruce Lee

As great and vibrant and excellent as someone else's life is, it will never be as good as the life you are living now. Even in the worst of circumstances, being you, being alive and having the opportunity of life, to make your own decisions of how to respond to situations, is the seed of greatness that may sprout into a life well lived.

Closing Question:

Who's your model of success in Health, Wealth, Love and Happiness?

How can you get closer to them?

What do you see in them that you see in yourself?

What are three steps you can take today to get closer to being more of who you desire to be?

Chapter 4:

On Influence

"What if our real ability to be truly influential is our ability to be influenced?"
—Unknown

Influence is everywhere. It affects everyone yet is predominantly in the hands of a small percentage of people. Why is that? It's available to everyone. There are people of influence of every culture, creed, and gender who inspire and evoke action across unrelated fields and interests. It's in every facet of our lives including nature and non-living organisms.

How influence penetrates our lives is what this chapter will explain. Here are the categories of influence:

- External
  0 People
  0 Environment

- Internal
  - 0   Self

- Verbal
  - 0   Spoken word

- Non-Verbal
  - 0   Body Language

External influence is concerned with the people around us. Family, coworkers, friends, teammates, and enemies. Second, the environment being geography, work space, and our homes. Internal influence is concerned with the inner self, the mind and our ability to exert control over our appetites, desires, reactions and impulses. It's the development of habit patterns that will run effortlessly so we may focus our energy on worthy struggles. Attention is one of the most valuable resources we have. Influence directs attention. Attention is energy and if you can capture someone's attention, you can capture their power.

> "Where you place your attention, is
> where you place your energy."
> —Dr. Joe Dispenza

This could be why women love attention so much...jokes aside, **influence has one primary purpose: to communicate ideas, feelings and moods in order to win a response.**

It's to make our audience think, feel, act, believe, vote, buy. It's also to make our environment cater to us as we adapt to it.

The first line of influence we have is our outward appearance. How we look- athletic or tired, preppy or haggard, tall and thin, short and heavy set, clean or dirty within an appropriate context determines how we are initially judged. If you are dressed in a suit for yard work, you may be judged a fool. This can be changed of course but non-verbally we size up the people we meet to see if they are a potential mate, client, friend or foe. It's our primitive brain circuits working to protect us and find opportunity. It's been said, when we open our mouths, we tell the world who we are. It's in our tone, our choice of words, our choice of language and cadence that will either pull others toward us or repel them after their initial non-verbal impression.

Two Perspectives

How do you view getting people to respond in a particular way? If you view the elements of the world with an optimistic lens, you may be more prone to say "influence". If you have a negative bias, you may say "manipulation". Now you may be wondering what's the difference?

At the core of it, its character and intentions. The same result could be produced by either manipulation or influence because they are, in essence, the same thing. What differentiates the two is how the other person feels after leaving your presence and the reputation of the person with whom you are engaged with. Typically if you feel forced, lied to, or cheated in order to get a result, that's manipulation. If you feel good, inspired, motivated by positive thoughts and emotion to take action, that's influence. Both are subtle. If they are not, they both fail. As humans, we don't enjoy being imposed upon or forced to do things against our will. When this happens, instinctively we fight back, even when it's for our own good. Just ask the parents of teenagers or the person helping someone with an addiction. They may know it's in their best interest but acting on their own accord feels better, more gratifying and powerful.

The person feeling imposed upon may entertain the communicator's ideas for a moment or even be amused by them but they are rarely moved to the desired action by the person trying to influence and if the person speaking is aggressive without an established relationship of trust and credibility, most people reject and dismiss this person totally. We may not know why consciously but our instincts do. We sense in their gestures and tone their intent. **People of great influence are subtly disarming.**

> "To reveal art and conceal the
> artist is the art's aim."
> —Oscar Wilde

The communicators themselves are not the target of attention, neither are their ideas, thoughts or feelings. Their primary objective is the well-being and gain of the audience they are communicating with. Some of you may be thinking: "How would they know what's good for me?"

They listen keenly. They ask open-ended questions. They listen deeper with their eyes and their ears. People of influence may give you something before they receive anything from you to provoke a response. It's information they use to know if they are moving in the right direction. By listening, they seek to intentionally add value to others. They **seek to understand before being understood.** This enables them to be of service.

Influencers have two qualities from which other traits of importance stem:

- They can vocally communicate their ideas clearly with simplicity, often in a casual conversational way that adds value to the listener.
- They are deep listeners. When listening they maintain a steady awareness of the information and emotion coming from their speaker and a poised stillness that lets you know they are with you.

So which comes first? Speaking or listening?

Depends. As a general rule:

Listening.

If you are going to speak, ask open-ended questions.

Why? (Open-ended)

Because that starts and then directs the conversation. More importantly, it leads to further conversation. It leaves room for someone to express more than a simple "yes", "no", "it was good" or "it was okay". Open-ended questions give the person you're with permission to dig deeper and share more of their thoughts and feelings, more of who they are or want to be.

Scientists have found that questions comprise approximately 6% of conversations, yet will generate approximately 60% of ensuing discussions.

Questions are the kindle that starts and keeps the fire of conversation going. It makes things interesting. We are dynamic, always changing and questions help open the door of uncovering what has changed, what is changing and what we like or dislike about it. We then can find out what to do about it and move closer together physically, mentally and emotionally. Thus, becoming more trusting and influential with this person or those people.

> "The character of the speaker is the most powerful of all means of influence."
> —Sarett Fostin

Are there other forms of communication? Of course. One of them is writing but writers, even though they are great communicators, speaking and listening are usually done in person. Speaking reaches everyone who understands the language immediately, even those who are illiterate and those who are foreign and are listening to the communicator in person, can usually understand the main idea of the message through body language and tone. It also is apparent the character and discipline this person has developed, because in order to speak well, clearly and confidently, one must know what they will say without edits. Even if they have practiced hundreds of hours, as they stand before us they are fluid, effortless in real time. It is who they have become or embodied and it's here in front us now unfolding as a life experience. As technology increases, email and texting have become more pronounced but it's supplemental. Speaking face to face, making eye contact with another human being has a deep significance that cannot be replaced without negative consequence to either party. Technology sustains connections that happen face to face and creates anticipation for those not met yet but unless there is face to face, in person contact, there will always be a void, a disconnect.

Listen Linda, Linda Listen.

When you let the other talk while you listen, you now know what they know, as well as what you know. If the person or people you are engaged with just ramble and complain and you're not stranded in a lifeboat with them, or dependent on them, politely walk away or direct their attention to another task. You do this by asking simple questions as Jordan Harbinger, founder of the Art of Charm Podcast, did when he and his friend were kidnapped and interrogated by Bosnian Agents of the state while traveling, working for the U.S government. Being that he was in a war-torn country, danger and conflict lurked everywhere. The people who kidnapped them were guards that were poorly trained, usually high on drugs such as meth and known to be violent and unethical when handling foreigners. After a brief confrontation, they brought Jordan and his friend back to the "safe house."

> "...back at their safe house...my friend is getting his ass beat. And I'm keeping extremely calm. On the outside. On the inside, I'm freaking out of course. But on the outside I'm staying as calm as humanly possible..the takeaway here is not just Keep Calm and Carry On when things are out of control. The takeaway here is you can control a situation by controlling your own emotions. Or your appearance of emotions.

And so, what this looked like in practice was that since this guy was angry, and getting upset and freaking out, and wired, **I was asking very logical questions.** 'Cause it's very difficult for your brain to have an extreme emotional reaction and also think about something logically at the same time.

...So I'm confusing them a little bit, but not with totally random stuff. With logical conversation...I started to talk about things like food, restaurants, light levels of politics that weren't going to get me in trouble. Areas around town. The logistics of travelling through their country. Driving laws. Just really, really concrete, logical topics."

There's always a way to better influence the situation in your favor and it begins with how you approach the situation. Begin with calmness, focus and questions, then listen like your life depends on it because it might. For those who want to genuinely connect and build stronger relationships, there are ways of listening that are better than others. Let's cover some best practices.

Traits of Influencers

Better called active listening, listening is an art that takes **practice, focus and patience.** While someone is giving you information you are simultaneously comprehending their words and gestures, while also empathizing and acknowledging you are with them through your gestures.

People who are the most attractive, and not just sexually speaking, but most pleasurable to be around, who begin receiving trust and building deep relationships are the people who:

- Make eye contact
- Ask for clarification
- Have poised body language
- Have open body language
- Smile and raise eyebrows
- Physical touch when appropriate
- Mirror body language subtly
- Use acknowledgement statements
- Give undivided attention
- Refrain from interruption and encourage the speaker to tell them more
- Use their language or vocabulary when appropriate
- Identify their insecurities and create inner security within them
- Become good storytellers
- Talk straight

- Communicate challenge
- Don't sell past the close
- Follow up and follow through

Let's unpack each of these.

Eye contact is important for many reasons. One it holds attention. The eyes let us know that the person listening and the person we are speaking to are with us. It creates the psychological feeling of connection. It's a soft gaze of about 5-8 seconds and then looking at other areas such as their mouth and back to the eyes to keep rapport. Eye contact between individuals also stimulates the release of oxytocin, the hormone we discussed in chapter two on love that chemically bonds individuals and deepens relationships. The eyes are also thought to emit energy.

Ever feel like someone is watching you? Their gaze, their energy was signaling you, vying for your attention or it could be alerting you of potential danger. It's been said that the eyes are the window to our soul and I believe that to be true. We can read a person's character, their intent through their eyes and know with a high degree of accuracy if this person or people we are engaged with are understanding us, moved by us or are disengaged. At the worst their eyes may indicate malevolence and anger. The eyes help us navigate and understand the person in front of us.

Ask for clarification means your asking them a follow question such as:

- So what you mean is…?

- What do you mean when you say…?

- Could you be more specific?

This gives them a chance to guide you and lead. In this way they get to further express themselves and their way of operating. When you come through with their technique, their way of doing something they feel as if they have influence and in turn you will have earned more influence with them, unless they are what I call a " user and abuser." Their eyes and actions over time will let you know if that's true or not and if they are of poor character, and you're continuing to be involved with them, then you will be in serious trouble without help at some time in the future.

From Marcus Aurelius:

To expect bad men not to do wrong is madness. For he who expects this desires an impossibility and to allow men to behave so to others and to expect them not to do you any wrong is irrational and tyrannical.

Deal with good people and your influence will be appreciated and move farther.

Poised body language means your body faces them. You're making eye contact with raised eyebrows that signal interest. If you are standing, your feet point towards them, your hands are in a relaxed position, and can be in your pockets with thumbs out which displays confidence. You're attentive, not looking around the room or playing with other items such as the phone, food, or utensils. If you are seated, again your feet are planted on the floor facing the speaker, your hands are visible and in a relaxed position, you're still and may nod your head slowly to let them know you are still with them as they talk.

Open body language means your arms are uncrossed, legs, feet or knees are pointed toward the speaker. Your hands are in a relaxed position where they can see them. It's been said that open hand gestures began in ancient times to show that no weapons were being concealed. I believe the logic is the same now. Again, all this goes within context. If someone is outside and it's cold they may cross their arms to keep warm. They may appear defensive but are still listening. If a woman is wearing a dress she may cross her legs out of courtesy and respect to herself but still have her foot or knee pointed towards you indicating positive interest. Read the environment and the situation before making a judgement.

Smile and raised eyebrow is what it sounds like. Try it in the mirror. I'll wait.

I mean it. Do it. If you have, you look interested, yes? Now try it with a blank face, what some women know as RBF: Resting Bitch Face. Not so inviting eh? The smile is disarming so long as it's not a morbid conversation or something that needs to be addressed seriously. Again influence is within context. Raised eyebrows signal "I'm interested and available. I'm safe and mean no harm." Most noticeable in adults, if you see wrinkled foreheads, it's likely they are open minded people. Those tight smooth foreheads may be more challenging and stubborn. Beware. Check for wrinkles next to the eyes when they smile. For someone who is faking this, they won't appear. A natural smile creates wrinkles by the eyes or "crows feet". False people only smile with their mouth.

Physical Touch when appropriate. Trust must be established first. When meeting someone, shake hands. That begins building trust. Depending on the country and the customs, a hug, holding hands or an arm around the shoulder, will create rapport. Gender will also be a factor in touch. If you are a male, other males will usually find it acceptable to pat one another on the shoulder or back or fist bump once you get to know them. Once you have gotten to know a female, a hug is usually more common than a handshake and if sitting in an interview a light tough of the knee or forearm is typically acceptable.

Mirrored body language will occur when you are in agreement or are in coherence with the person speaking. This usually happens subconsciously but can be brought to conscious awareness without much effort. If you are too obvious about it, it can be offensive as if you are mocking the other person rather than mirroring them. It's very subtle.

Acknowledgement statements are phrases such as:

- I agree.

- Right on.

- Thank you for sharing that. You always inspire me.

- I love how open and honest you are.

- I love talking to you and sharing insights.

They usually happen at the end of a conversation but can happen when you agree with them as they speak. They let the other person know you find them valuable and you value the relationship and are on the same page. In the best selling book, *How to Win Friends and Influence People* by Dale Carnegie, one of the most repeated reminders when communicating with others is the phrase "Be lavish in your praise and hearty in your approbation." It makes people feel good about what they do, say and who they are. When you make people feel good in those ways they are inclined to want to do the same for you but more importantly, to do that for others they meet outside your interactions.

Undivided Attention is attention that is whole. You stop what you are doing to listen. It's focused solely on the person you are engaged with as if nothing else exists. It's not staring without blinking or not moving. It's alertness and poise that's natural, it's in essence drawing you in to listen. It's how you would look if something was important, interesting and you wanted to learn more.

Refrain from interruption and encourage them to tell you more. This is tough, yet creates strong connections very quickly. When someone is telling you something, something good, something bad, go deep into it. **Find out why it's important to them.** Don't try to one up them with something you have done or been through. That only makes them feel unheard and unimportant. Even if it *feels* unimportant to you, it *is* important to them and that's what matters and they want to share it. By sharing, they are trying to connect and if trust and influence is what you are trying to establish, then it would be in your best interest to understand them. They will feel more connected as a result and feel compelled to be around you more.

Use their language. If they use certain phrases or words, also use them so you become relatable so long as it's not offensive or harmful to them or others in your environment. The person talking will feel you understand and feel connected. If it's another language like Spanish, for example, and you know how to speak it fluently, speak in their mother tongue. It will create an air of exclusiveness between each of you.

Identify their insecurities and create an inner security within them. We all have our weak spots. To point them out, particularly if unwarranted or before trust is established will usually destroy any chances of connection. Our insecurities come out in all kinds of unspoken ways, usually fairly obvious to outside observers and when identified, keep them to yourself then create inner security within them. The confidence and positivity you evoke will bring each of you closer together.

Become a good story teller. Leaders, people of great influence all tell compelling stories. Just like we spoke of in chapter one, stories and narratives is how we think. We identify with stories deeply. The right story can inspire action, can inspire a movement and change the way people think for the better. This was the difference between someone like Cicero and Demosthenes in Ancient Greece. Both were renowned as being great orators. The difference was after a speech from Cicero people were entertained.

After a speech from Demosthenes, people were moved to take action.

Talk straight and tell the truth tactfully. Speak from facts mixed with measured emotions. Exaggeration is usually a sign of lack of self worth and wanting to inflate something to make it more than it really is. When people do that and we find out it's not true, respect is lost and with it, influence. Jim Rohn said it well, "The truth will set you free. Free to do what? Amend your errors and set up new disciplines."

Communicate challenge. When we offer a challenge to someone, we raise them up a level. We without saying it directly, communicate they are capable of more and believe in them. Through adversity, we form deeper bonds.

Don't sell past the close. When we overload people with information in an effort to help them and discharge our knowledge, we push them away and can make them feel less about themselves and make ourselves appear egotistical and spastic. The person listening only needs enough to take action and convince themselves. French Poet, Anatole France phrased this well: "Do not try to satisfy your vanity by trying to teach a great many things. Awaken people's curiosity. It's enough to open minds; do not overload them. Put there just a spark. If there is some good inflammable stuff, it will surely set fire."

Follow up and follow through after you have met or spoken to one another. Depending on the relationship, call them, text them or email them saying:

- Hey brother, it was really great catching up. Let's get together again soon. I always enjoy your company.

- Hey girl, I had such a great time connecting with you. I love our talks and keeping up to date. Let's go out this weekend if you are free.

- Thanks again for a great time today. Your energy is so revitalizing and refreshing. Looking forward to connecting again.

If this interaction has been via letter, text, email or video before you meet and you say you are going to do something, **do it.** Doing what you say establishes trust, credibility and puts you in alignment with your values and potentially their values as well. You will maintain your integrity and increase the weight of your words which affects your level of influence.

Crab People

No, not the South Park episode. Get that out of here. What I'm talking about is the Maryland blue crab and how people can be just like them. For those of you who are unfamiliar, the Maryland blue crab is a delicacy and is revered for its sweet meat, the thrill of being on the bay and is associated with family, festivity and fun in the summer. I highly suggest you come to Kent Island and try some.

If you have never caught them, they are quite wiley, especially if you are using a trot line. They can be quite large, sometimes 9" across and with large claws to pinch, they grab ahold of anything trying to get in their way. Typically when caught they are placed into a wooden basket. Once in the basket with other crabs they will fight, sometimes literally ripping the claws off other crabs right out of their sockets and off their shells.

If one crab starts to make its way to the top of the basket and climb out, the others pull it back down and fight again. That's why many times someone crabbing will leave the top off the basket because the other crabs will prevent the ones on top from escaping until the basket is full to the brim.

What brings them to mind in relation to people and influence is that when you begin to climb higher in your life, begin doing well and finding success, a lot of people around you won't like that.

Why?

It's a dark aspect of human nature. It's how the average person is. Success to some becomes a spotlight that shines down on their missed opportunities.

People, particularly the people closest to you may comment, slander or begin to throw shade upon your actions and achievements. Your winning makes them feel insufficient. It's not that you are actually doing this. It's a reflection of themselves and their failures and where they came up short and didn't revisit the darkness and transform it into a win. They will try to drag you back down with them, into the basket, into the unnecessary discomfort of the status quo.

And just like the crab, seeking its way back home, into the bay, into freedom, you must seek your own freedom, aware that people will try to pull you back into the norm, to where they feel comfortable with you and believe you belong. They will try to influence you to be on their team or their path. If that path or those people are not part of your plan, just keep climbing. They may try to verbally tear you limb from limb, fight you..let it go and move forward.

As you gain more clout and influence, they may change and support you again. Once more, move forward. **Set the example and make the best of the situation.** This is the beginning of leadership.

> "Leadership is influence."
> —John C. Maxwell

Final Thoughts

The takeaway here is **listen**. Ask open ended questions and listen some more. Be tactfully authentic in your responses and behavior. Save your story and find out more about theirs. What is important to this person?

Identify their insecurities privately and create a feeling of inner security within them. Find where they have been and where they want to go. What has been and what currently is a landmark moment, a pivot point for them, a point of realization?

Make eye contact and be with this person. Though it's only for a moment, those moments linger and ripple into other relationships. Be aware of the consciousness you bring to the environment you enter.

Closing Questions:

What five people are you around most?

Why?

What makes them valuable to you?

What are they doing around you?

Who is winning in areas you also desire to win?

How can you learn more about them and their process?

CHAPTER 5:

ON LEADERSHIP

"Leadership is everything. You show me
anything that wins and I'll show you a
leader at work."
—Arthur O. Williams

_____

A Leader of Leaders

WE BEGIN WITH conflict, for if there was peace, there
would be no story, nor would there be a need for a leader. At
the beginning of time before the world was created, Tiamat,
the goddess of the sea, the mother of everything and Apsu,
the god of freshwater were locked in an embrace. Tiamat
and Apsu represent chaos and order, masculine and feminine, and through their union, give rise to the other gods.

Tiamat being the mother of everything and creator of
the other gods, felt deep love for her creations. These other
gods though disturbed Apsu. They kept him up at night
and distracted him from his work during the day. Because

of this he decides one day to eliminate these gods, to kill them. Horrified, Tiamat tells her eldest son, Enki, the god of Wisdom of Apsu's plan. Enki thinks of the best possible course of action and puts Apsu into a deep sleep, so deep in fact, it kills him. From his remains, Enki created part of the earth.

Upon hearing of the death of Apsu, Tiamat becomes enraged. She did not anticipate this outcome. In her rage she decides that perhaps it is time for the gods to be slayed. In order to make this a reality, she assembles a battalion of chimeric monsters. In charge of these beasts is Kingu, what today would be equivalent to Satan. As each god goes out to confront Tiamat and resolve matters, they are defeated and cast away by her. Her mind is made up. Kingu begins to slay the other gods, winning in every battle.

Whatever these elder gods' powers are, they are not what can confront chaos and create order. Something more is needed. Then one day after the elder gods have been continually beaten back by Tiamat, a young god named Marduk emerges. Marduk is unique compared to that of the other gods in that he has eyes all the way around his head and he can speak magic words. He has the ability to speak day into night and night into day and he can see in all directions simultaneously.

Seeing the potential of this god, the elder gods inform him of the situation with Tiamat. With little debate Marduk is elected to step forward and try his hand in stopping the actions of the Mother Goddess. He accepts this challenge and does so on one condition only: That the other gods follow him, declare him the god of gods and allow him to declare all destinies.

Believing him capable, the gods accept this proposition.

Before he goes to confront Tiamat, he gathers a net and summons the wind. Upon encountering Tiamat, Marduk fills her with a wind and captures her in the net. This is how he encapsulates chaos itself. Once captured in the net, Marduk cuts Tiamat into pieces and from those pieces he creates the rest of the world left undone by Enki. He then defeats the army of monsters including Kingu. From the blood of Kingu, Marduk creates human beings to inhabit the world and serve the gods.

In Mesopotamia, where the story originated, the Mesopotamian people would go outside their walled city in celebration of the New Year. Leaving the order of the city into the untamed nature outside the city walls symbolized leaving order and confronting chaos. They would bring statues representing the gods and act this story line out. The current emperor, who was believed to be the human manifestation of Marduk, would be forced to kneel before the people without his royal clothing and then was beaten with a glove. He was asked where he had failed as a "Marduk" that previous year and how he will improve in the upcoming year. He would recount his inadequacies in confronting chaos. After this ritual they would continue the enactment having Marduk win. The king would then have sex with a with a royal prostitute, a benefit of a king which is represented in confronting chaos and from which order can be extracted from the experience. In essence that would be a new life, a child, the organization of elements to create a human being, a consciousness.

This ancient story, though outdated in many ways, has elements that continue to stand the test of time of what we need, value and define as a leader. This is what the Mesopotamian people were trying to figure out. Who or what was king of the gods? Who leads leaders? Who can confront chaos then create or restore order? In more modern terms what defines leadership?

Leadership defined is the capacity to see what is going on around you and the ability to use your language properly in a transformative manner to turn chaos into order. This type of leadership was also used by the ancient Greeks. They believed that if one was to be a leader of people, they had to become a master of language. Not just the spoken word but in how they moved as well. They had to **understand human nature and body language.**

Now some of you may be wondering about humans being created from the blood of a terrible monster. What does being created from the monster Kingu mean?

It means that as humans we have the capacity to deceive, to be evil and malevolent. We can twist reality. Humans are the only known animal that can willingly deceive with the intent to hurt others. Just because someone acts good and benevolent doesn't mean they are good. We have to understand human nature. We have to learn to lead ourselves. We are not perfect and with that known fact, we can choose a better way of being. We can act properly and just. We know that we will fail from time to time but we can choose to confront that chaos and create order or find someone who will.

In following a leader and their plans we must still observe and make our own decisions. If we follow a bad plan, that's our own fault. We must learn to see deception and danger then avoid it. It's up to us to communicate information to our leaders and people before it happens, even when we feel fear. That's part of confronting chaos and restoring order.

Follow to Lead

> "I must follow them, I am their leader."
> —Basic Principles of Speech

Why do people follow? Most people are like sheep. They follow the first dominant voice on the scene. A few reasons are that that person appears willing to take responsibility for their actions and the group and is confident of themselves and their ability. As individuals, we want that same ability in our own lives and by being near them and under their guidance, we may obtain some of that or at least be taken care of and protected. That's not always true though, particularly in a time now where social media distorts and twists the reality of a person's life.

True leaders who create a following are those who are doing the right things—turning chaos into order, finding solutions and helping the group—so we may learn, then as a result of their leadership, lead others around us in the future, repeating this positive cycle of leaders creating leaders. In relation to parenting, you wouldn't want your kid to follow your rules, your instruction because it's what you said but so they will learn, become autonomous and begin living on their own terms without your supervision in a way that is useful to society and future generations. The point isn't to raise a child but to cultivate an adult.

Otherwise, that kid will grow up biologically as an adult but will have to rely on others and need assistance for everything, adding an unnecessary strain to the parents and to society. This goes for training people at work, in sports, and just giving advice. At first the feeling of leading and having the answers for someone can feel rewarding, like you're needed and special. At that moment you are. This person or the people you are with need someone and you happen to be there. That superior position though, is a very small part of being a leader and should be short lived, as in they need to learn to handle situations through training and information they gather from you when things go south. The second part is you have more to learn from them, sometimes they may lead you into unfamiliar territory. Let the situation unfold a moment before objecting. It's a give and take relationship at times. In a word, humility.

Letting go after demonstrating and guiding, can be tougher for the leader than for the trainee but there comes a time when the person being trained, coached or in need of help needs to fail, try again and lead their own way. The leader may need to offer emotional support and encouragement during that time but they know by giving the information to the trainee, employee or student and stepping back they offer them respect and in a way, say "I believe you are tough enough to handle this challenge." This also helps develop strength, respect and confidence in the person performing. After they have overcome their struggle, you may see eye to eye and operate more as equals than as teacher and student in this arena.

"Never above you, never below you,
always beside you."
—Sgt. Brian Jacklin

The word *lead* is derived from the ancient Hebrews meaning to be out in front, to drive. What does it mean to be out in front driving? It means doing what needs to be done and doing it first. Being the example, an exemplar. Leaders are the ones who unify people around a larger vision, a cause or a mission. Steve Jobs is a prime example of someone who had a large vision and inspired people to join him.

In the beginning days of Apple, and learning about programming, Jobs would go out and find the best people to do the tasks he wasn't very good at. He aimed high. One of the people he called on was John Sculley, CEO of Pepsi. A tough sell considering this man was established in his profession and his life and was in essence asked to join a small startup compared to the behemoth drink company he was currently in charge of. Initially he rejected the young man and kept on about his business. Then one day after several talks, Jobs had enough and fired back with the famous comment that won Sculley over:

"Do you want to sell sugar water for the rest of your life? Or do you want to come with me and change the world?"

Not a way of communicating I recommend out the gate but with boldness, skills and the results Steve Jobs was producing, he won Scully over. This is an internal example, within the company of Apple but people around the world use the Apple products daily, defend the brand with their life and support the culture it inspires. In fact, this book and the other book I've written have been written on an IPhone. Besides being a great product, Jobs had a mindset that people matter, things don't or what they call in the Navy, "humans over hardware". He knew other programmers had made superior computers at the time, better than his but he knew how to gather people, get them working together on a single purpose and use their collective thinking to outperform others.

Negative Capability

This concept was introduced by English poet John Keats in 1817. Keats was trying to figure out what made Shakespeare so much more creative than other writers. He came to create the term negative capability. It's defined as **the ability to hold two opposing ideas in mind without being uncomfortable while pursuing a vision and embracing situations even when it leads to confusion, uncertainty and suspending judgement as possibilities surface while keeping an open mind to each possibility.** The greatest leaders in history and some of the ones you may know personally all have the ability to take action on what they believe, even when they are uncertain or what arises doesn't make sense at the moment and accept that there are many possible outcomes, yet work with the outcome that is coming into fruition.

> "The test of a first-rate intelligence is the ability to hold two opposed ideas in mind at the same time and still retain the ability to function."
> —F. Scott Fitzgerald

It's a mixture of experience and faith that drives them to continue on the path of unknown possibilities. Is negative capability a requisite to be a leader? No I don't believe it is. It's a trait that the best leaders have though.

Leading the Way

In Niccolò Machiavelli's book *The Prince*, he gives advice on how a prince should govern his state, himself and his militia.[118] In referring to taking care of the people of the city, he writes: "It is man's nature to obligate himself as much for the benefits he gives as for the benefits he receives." This means that when the people who defend the cause and the leader have been beaten, battered and their possessions destroyed, the people need to see their leader step up and help them rebuild what's been broken.

Sounds like common sense but it's not always the case. In an interview between Jocko Willink and Ssg. Dave Hall who served in Vietnam, they touched on aspects of good and bad leadership, in this particular example, they talk about bad leadership. Hall believed in order to lead he had to be a participant in the tough times with his men. If they were unloading material, he would unload material. If his men had to bathe in a bomb crater, he would too. So long as what they were doing didn't compromise his ability to see the larger perspective of the mission or plan, he was essentially just another soldier. One of the stories Hall shares was after weeks of leading and fighting alongside his men, he asked all the men in his platoon to fill and load sandbags to create a barrier and set up a new perimeter for camp, in which he was also participating. Then from the tent near where the platoon was, his Colonel caught wind of Hall helping and called him aside:

"You see that shade over there?" Said the Colonel.

Hall answered back "yeah."

"Go sit down over there and watch your guys fill sandbags."

"But Sir, these guys are part of me." Said Hall.

"Doesn't matter. Sit in the shade and watch them do it."

Hall looked back with disbelief.

"If you want to fill sandbags I can make it so you can do that." The Colonel said with an air cockiness.

"No, sir, that's okay."

Hall had to go back out to tell his men what he now had to do and having built some leadership capital with his men, they understood. He took the hit so he could continue to lead his men and continue with forward progress once his commanding officer left the field. The other sergeants were either dying or finding ways to hide while their men were in harm's way. Dying because of poor decision making and lack of group cohesion.

The benefits of a leader may be greater than that of whom they are leading but so are the consequences when things go wrong. The position of a leader represents someone who can bear the burden better and for sustained periods of time, while also thinking farther ahead and more clearly under pressure than the people he is leading in this particular arena. It is known that the leader has more responsibility and gets more pay, more rewards and benefits but it's an unwritten law that they take the fault for failures, for defeat, and are obligated to the people to get them on the correct path whatever the cost is to the leader, which in the case of a prince or a military leader, could be their life.

> "It is a king's business to do good
> and be abused for it."
> —Marcus Aurelius

That sort of consequence in the day to day of the average man or woman is unlikely, though many moms and dads would agree they would give their lives to save their children. But that cost may come in the form of standing up for your people and what you believe and losing your job. It may mean being cut from the team or dropped from the program. It may mean working later hours with your team to make up for the mistakes created by them from lack of communication. At any rate, the leader is to serve the people and act in their best interests. When they do, the people will more than likely step up when things get tough.

A Centaur, A Prince and A Warrior

When Achilles was a young boy, his mother brought him to Centaur Chiron, a half man, half beast to be trained and disciplined. He learned not just about war and combat. He learned how to be measured, tactful and understanding amongst the people.

To be totally in one and not contain any of the other is to be unbalanced. People will be in fear of one and abusive to the other. Leaders must adapt to their environment and ascertain rhythms in between if they are to lead and win. As men and women today, I believe this means we must be aware of and use both natures. Be both savage and saint or lion and fox, as Machiavelli once said, because "the lion cannot defend against the snares and the fox cannot defend against the wolves. Together they root out and terrify the opposition."

Sometimes we must be hard not only on ourselves but also with those we love, we must yell and howl until our message connects. We must destroy those things that stand in the way on our path. Evil is real and must be rooted out and transcended. Just as that's true, at other times we have to listen, nourish, be kind, mild and gentle with ourselves, with our team. We retreat to our place of comfort to lick our wounds to heal back stronger.

Savage and Saint, Lion and Fox, Alpha and Beta are intertwined. They, like Yin and Yang, play on each other's energy. Both are necessary for success. Find the ones who have been in wars, find the ones who know hurt and have used it as fuel to be kinder, wiser, smarter, and better. They have boons to bestow upon us.

A Warrior in the Garden

"A dog won't tolerate being treated too kindly and
neither will a man or woman."[120]
—Robert Greene

No one, not kids, not dogs, and especially women, don't like or respect a leader who is too kind and agreeable. Machiavelli in *The Prince*, says this well:

> "...For how one lives and how one ought to live are so far apart that he who spurns what is actually done for what ought to be done will achieve ruin rather than his own preservation."[119]

This means that one needs to see things as they are first, before they see them better than they are. **We must deal in reality if we are to be effective.** Otherwise, we build a house of cards upon a foundation of sand, which, when the foundation inevitably shifts, it all comes crashing down.

Machiavelli continues:

> "A man who strives to make a show of correct comportment in every circumstance can only come to ruin among so many who have other designs. Hence it is necessary for a prince who wishes to maintain his position to learn how to be able not to be good, and to use or not use this ability according to circumstances."

This translates to: know when to stay on the path but know when to break the rules. Frederick the Great understood this when he wrote: "A perfect person, like Plato's Republic does not exist, it is a figment of the imagination. It is not characteristic of human nature to produce beings exempt from human weakness and defects. The finest medallions have a reverse side."

We must train to handle the reverse side and recognize it in the side that is often most enjoyable.

Did you know the word "nice" is a derivative of a French word meaning to be foolish, not knowing, naïve, silly, or ignorant? People often mistake being kind for being nice but there is a major difference. Weak people are nice. Strong people are kind. Weakness is a lack of knowledge and will be taken advantage of. Strength is an awareness and choosing a positive, understanding attitude even when others are rude and disagreeable. Any leader who is nice, will be dethroned or worse lead his people to slaughter.

A kind leader is one who, knowing his people, his opposition and terrain, gives and acts benevolently because he chooses to, even though he is dangerous and seeks to make peace, though is intelligently, resourcefully and willingly ready to make war.

"The best men I know are dangerous."
—Jordan B. Peterson

There is an anecdote that I believe characterizes a leader:

One day a master and his disciple were walking side by side through a beautiful garden. The master mentions how peaceful the garden is amongst the early morning air and how this time of national peace is good. Pondering over his latest lesson from the master, the disciple suddenly stops and asks: "Master, now you talk about and preach to me the ways of peace. Yet after many years of combat training and mental conditioning I have learned from you deadly techniques of combat and the tactics of war. How do you reconcile the two?" The master gracefully squats, chooses a flower and plucks it. "My disciple: it is better to be a warrior tending to his garden than a gardener in a war."

"To be prepared for war is one of the most effective means of preserving peace."
—George Washington

A true leader is one who is a warrior in the garden, not a gardener in a war. They are peaceful people who are ready for conflict, situationally aware and able to defend themselves and the people they care about most. This means that to grow as a leader, one must become dangerous by embracing danger, training hard physically, and training hard mentally by reading and studying human nature as well as the aspects of their domains.

The Law of Irreducible Rascality

To think everyone, including our most powerful leaders in the world, are all good and virtuous would be a fault. We are human, we make mistakes. We are not gods but we are divine. At the worst people can be genocidal and by no means am I saying it is okay to be bad or malevolent but it's reality. Some people call those darker parts their demons, Plato called it the "dark horse", Goethe called it his "daemon". Identifying our dark elements, becoming aware of them, allows us to transcend that side of our nature and use it to our advantage. Many leaders can be rascals and it adds to their character. Alan Watts, the American-British zen philosopher uses the analogy of a soup with no salt in it. A man or woman who is portrayed as all good or does all good is dry, banal, has no flavor, no zest. Salt in a large quantity ruins the meal but in a small quantity is delightful.

"So everyone has to be salted with a certain amount of unrespectability. Otherwise they are impossible and intolerable, but as a fervent cook, don't overdo it."

Someone who is all serious all the time sucks the joy of life out of work and play. Someone who is playful all the time is too gullible and immature. It's the balance of each at the proper time that produces an irresistible charismatic character. It's been said that one is not truly an expert until they can handle serious subjects with a light touch, a sense of humor and communicate it with simplicity so anyone can grasp its concepts.

Selfish and Selfless

How does a leader serve his people?

I believe there are two elements:

- Selfishness
- Self-lessness

It may come as a surprise to you that leaders are selfish. Many women, particularly moms, will understand this more than men I believe. The reason I put selfishness on here is that in order to be in surplus, gather an abundance of resources, get adequate rest, and even time for yourself, one has to be selfish for a while.

> "I spent the first half of my life making money
> and the second half of my life giving it away to do
> the most good and the least harm."
> —Andrew Carnegie

Growing up this is how we start off. Selfish, self-centered and thinking the world revolves around us because, in essence, as a baby and toddler, it does. This, if prolonged, becomes a negative selfishness. Then as we grow older and mature, we come to realize the need to give away things that we don't need or use to someone else who could use them. That could be in the form of time, energy, knowledge, a listening ear, clothes, tools, ect. Then instead of gathering things because we believe them useful for just us, we accumulate knowledge, skills, money, and insight so we may be of greater utility to those around us when called upon. This is what is known as positive selfishness.

Where does this positive selfishness come from?

This positive type of selfishness grows out of an accurate understanding of what we need to do and who we need to become in order to maximize our utility for others. It emanates from a sense of how we should develop our abilities, get ourselves into the right state of body and mind, and organize our thoughts and feelings so that they can one day be useful to the people we encounter. If we don't get to bed early, eat well, study and practice, save our money and invest it wisely and love ourselves, take care of our needs, how would we be able to serve others who are in need? The answer: we wouldn't. It's the same reason they say to put the oxygen mask on yourself first in the event of an airplane crash before helping someone else near you. **We're only as good to someone as we are good to ourselves.**

Many people confuse those who are positively selfish with the mean-spirited, cold hearted and self interested. Read the person and view their actions over time, inquire a bit because it could be just that but if the person has a track record of helpfulness and is verbal about their motives and their actions align, it's likely true they want to be of greater service. The key is learning to persuasively convey the message that we are not being callous but will simply better serve those around us by not operating in the status quo for a while. Those who don't understand, don't need to understand. Block out the naysayers, the doubters and keep working diligently in your own way until the results are irrefutable. You act for a higher purpose rather than just for yourself and produce desired results that affect you and everyone around you positively. You are making being in that space better. By acting in this way, we avoid becoming an inconvenience to others and avoid what is only on the surface a good idea: always putting other people first.

The second and more familiar way people may think of leaders is selflessness. Defined as being more concerned with the needs of others than one's own needs. Good parents are like this for their children. True leaders are like this for their organizations. They have reservoirs of strength, knowledge, physical, mental, emotional and financial energy that when one or multiple of the team members are down, they can help pick up the slack usually with what seems like minimal cost to the leader but may cost them everything. The leader still acts despite the cost to themselves for the greater good of the mission, cause and purpose.

> "The one who plants trees, knowing he will never sit in their shade, has at least started to understand the meaning of life."
> —Rabindranath Tagore

Soldiers are well known for giving their life for their comrades and country. Michael Monsoor, is a prime example. A young man at the age of 25, serving as an active SEAL jumped on a grenade to save two of his team members while under attack by insurgents on September 29, 2006. More commonly though, you may witness a mother tending to the needs of her child giving up the last bit of her time to make sure they get to practice or are fed. One of your friends may take the day off to come and listen to an issue that's been gnawing away at you or you yourself might give something away you value because it serves a greater purpose other than yourself.

Self-lessness is learned and takes time to develop. It is not innate like selfishness. As we grow more mature, we find greater value in people and relationships formed. The utility in objects and the joy of serving something greater than ourselves, be it a higher power such as God, an organization, a spouse and family, we begin to find it easier to let go of the idea of self or ego and the things associated with it and willingly sacrifice those things, knowing how much those around us will benefit, even when we are no longer in the picture. While we are still around though, and acting with a legacy in mind, we find our pleasure is multiplied because there's only one of us and billions of others. The more those around us are healthy, happy and winning, the more we will be too.

Dichotomy of Improvement

A common theme amongst most men and women who are leaders is their need to fix things. More so men outwardly and women inwardly but in general, there is a desire to make things better and solve problems. It makes the person leading feel as if they are serious and needed but one thing we must remember is that some problems will never be solved, some problems will never be "fixed". Does that mean we shouldn't try to solve problems?

No, I believe it means knowing the context and nature of the situation.

When something announces itself to you that is in need of repair, first see if you can fix it.

Ask:

How could I be of service?

Maybe you have a particular skill set that could aid the situation or you may listen well and can assemble information quickly, that may lead to a creative insight that may turn a problem into a product or a solution. There is a dichotomy here though. As a leader, you don't <u>need</u> to fix everything, even people and systems that are broken. We have to let those around us, particularly those who need something fixed, to try to solve the problem themselves.

Why?

They need the mental and emotional muscles that you have developed through struggle. If we don't give them a chance to fix something first, we weaken them and in an indirect way offer less respect than if we had given them the opportunity to solve the problem themselves. Training and guidance should be offered during this time but let the people or person think, experiment and attempt to figure out a solution.

When the systems and methods in place aren't working, like we discussed in chapter 3 on models, seek out people in places where things are already working. Likely the solution is to emulate that system, adjusting it to the needs of your situation and then multiply what's working across your domain.

- Where are people injured and still working?

- Who has had a broken relationship but is still loving?

- Who has had defeat but still found a way to win?

These people more than likely have the solutions we're looking for. True leaders have the humility to accept solutions though it's not theirs. Getting the problem solved and their people taken care of is the main objective.

"Be part of the answer, not part of the problem."[126]
—Sgt. David Hall

Leaders look for ways to make things better. One reason most people fail to make things better is because they try to do it all at once, they think it all needs to be fixed right now and it overwhelms them. Rather the opposite is true. You have to start to begin. This means start small and begin doing something correctly towards the major initiative. It builds confidence and momentum for overcoming the next obstacle. An example many people can relate to is exercise. So you can only do 25 squats at once. The workout calls for 200 squats. Do sets of 25 until you can only do sets of 10 reps or even 1 rep. Small consistent wins over time will get you to the end result you desire. The same goes with a book, or school paper. It isn't all written in a day. We write a page or two or five. We do the best we can, offering quality work then we take a break and go again. Remember, Rome wasn't built in a day.

"How do you get a miracle going? Do all you can, do the best you can, rest very little."[128]
Jim Rohn

A simple question you may ask yourself when feeling overwhelmed is:

- How can I make this place better for just 30 minutes?

Begin there. Set a target. One step at a time we get ahead. We gradually see progress. Not as rewarding upfront but fulfilling and satisfying on the backend. And yes, you should celebrate small victories with small rewards. That builds confidence and momentum but it must be in proportion to the results achieved and it shouldn't be expected. **The result you were looking to achieve is the reward.**

> "Spend each day trying to be a little wiser than you were when you woke up. Discharge your duties faithfully and well. Step by step you get ahead, but not necessarily in fast spurts, but you build discipline by preparing for fast spurts. Slug it out one inch at a time, day by day and at the end of the day, if you live long enough, most people get what they deserve."
> —Charlie Munger

Slow progress, built with a solid foundation of fundamental skills tends to last longer, is sustainable and will withstand resistance from outside forces. You can also maintain control of situations because there is less to manage at once. You can handle one issue no problem, two issues, no big deal. But when you start getting several at a time, unnecessary friction builds and results in inaction or poor action. As novelist Anthony Trollope once wrote, "a small daily task, if it really be daily, will beat the labors of a spasmodic Hercules." The more efficient and skillful we become at a task, the less time we spend doing it, leaving room for the activities we truly enjoy.

About Questions

Do your coworkers constructively (or blatantly) question you often? How about your kids? Your spouse? Your friends?

If they do...good.

Why is that good? It gives you an opportunity to validate your actions and results. It keeps you sharp. If you don't have the answer, then maybe what you're doing is wrong or could be improved. We don't just win once and call ourselves reliable. We have to keep winning. When students question their teachers, when employees question their bosses and children question their parents, it's a way to explore the unknown and prove the known. Do we need faith and trust in our leaders? Of course. Nevertheless though, questions deepen understanding and questions open up avenues of new ways of performing tasks. It's the pinnacle of learning. When the people we are around question everything at the appropriate time, a wealth of knowledge and potential experience becomes available to everyone listening. Don't just accept things as they are, challenge it and find what's true then what to do about it.

> "Trust in Radical Truth
> and Radical Transparency."
> —Ray Dalio

This questioning will create disagreements at times. That's okay and should be welcomed. It's an opportunity to root out the ego, detach and discover the best course of action. Holding on to outdated methods and past routines because "that's the way it's always been done" is a poor reason and will eventually lead to rigidity and staleness, ultimately ending in the end of a relationship, a team or business. Keeping an open mind, sharing tactfully what's on yours and discussing the positive and negative consequences of proposals allows for stronger cohesion to develop among members of the team and deeper insights to be readily utilized.

A question to ask yourself before a meeting, before an event, or a phone call is:

What outcome do I want? And why?

If you are in a group:

What outcome do we want? And why?

When you know the outcome you want and why it's important, the steps to getting there become clearer and the why gives you energy to persevere through obstacles. Once outcomes are clear, execution becomes the next right thing to do. As you execute, morale will improve and with it results.

> "To know the right thing to do,
> and not do it, is weakness."
> —Confucius

Check Yourself Before You Wreck Yourself

I first heard the term PMA, positive mental attitude used by Napoleon Hill in one of his recorded lectures and would later hear of it used in different ways by people who are considered highly successful and people in professions that demand clear thinking while working with groups of hostile people or dangerous situations.

Our attitude on the day to day may seem insignificant. Sure our friends may want space to "get away", our coworkers avoidant in the afternoon or our spouse may just decide they want space but whether we get hyped up or stay calm while things go wrong or when something doesn't go our way can determine the outcome of our relationships, income, and status at home, at work and in public. In the most extreme cases, the wrong attitude could kill you.

"Attitude development is the key to everything."
—Sgt. Jim Webb

Anger, frustration, rage, all serve purposes. They're known as "tools of last resort". It's the tool we use when all else has failed repeatedly. On most every occasion though, the attitude of calm, confidence and control of bodily and emotional responses is the answer. Laurence Gonzales, thrill seeker, pilot and author explains in his book, *Deep Survival*, elements of skill, attitude, and humility that separates who lives, who dies and why.

In the appendix there is a Rules of Adventure and a list of 12 things survivors do well. I won't cover them all here but three major ones among all people who survive is 1) calmness under pressure. They stay logical or use emotion to channel logical thinking. 2) A sense of humor, typically dark humor and 3) an attitude of never giving up. Once in the thick, they come to terms with reality and do whatever it takes to get home.

I encourage you to read this book for its life lessons and the fascinating look into the psychology of people under stress but the three elements mentioned above will help us navigate the day to day interactions with those around us at home, at work and in public. Let's unpack these three items a bit more.

People can be everything we wish they weren't and we are no different. What separates the leaders from the herd is their ability to manage their responses while still carrying the responsibility of their well-being and the well being of the group. When we are stressed, be it from a workout, a written test, a confrontation at work or in public, the body floods with chemicals called catecholamines adrenaline and norepinephrine.

Released from the adrenal medulla, adrenaline acts primarily on the lungs, skeletal muscles and arteries through alpha and beta receptors. In short, it prepares the body for action, either fight or flight. Norepinephrine is very similar but only acts on alpha receptors. It is released by the brain structure called the locus coeruleus. Though comparatively small in number in the brain, noradrenergic neurons project into many other areas of the brain and spinal cord. Norepinephrine functions to increase alertness, keeping us vigilant for more on coming threats and escape routes, enhances the formation and retrieval of short and long term memories and enhances the activity in the prefrontal cortex as well as other brain regions. A study done at Stanford University found that, **when we experience stressful events, our brain also secretes DHEA, a neurosteroid that helps our brains grow, recover and gain new knowledge from the experience.**[130] Stress, either from the mundane to significant, is a guide helping us to act quickly and stay aware of such events in the future.

The cardiovascular system that carries these hormones are also affected differently when stress arises and how we think about stress, either a challenge or threat, will change the dilation of our blood vessels. In each case our heart is still pounding but when we experience stress negatively our blood vessels constrict. If that happens often, we are susceptible to heart attack and heart disease, a common death in the US and among type A personalities or "hard chargers". When we experience stress positively though, the blood vessels stay wide open and relaxed, allowing more blood flow. This positive response is the same as when someone feels joyful or is acting courageously.

Many young men and women understand this in a physical way, yet it takes time to transfer this felt experience into thought and concrete information that can be used in other domains. I learned a majority of this first in the gym, then began studying and researching the experiences and how they related. Once I was working full time, I saw how they could transfer into business and relationships.

Through weight training, endurance training, being able to do hard things and handle hurt physically, emotionally or mentally are all symbols to being a strong leader. They are indicators of a strong person. Just like one who exercises a strong will or excellent decision making is likely a person of excellence because their habits show it. It is usually not the thing itself but what you are doing. For example, a heavy squat does not make you a good leader or a good person but that you are able to handle high stress and perform well and stay calm, confident and in control of your body and emotions, that makes you a good leader. The activity may differ but the response will be the same. As a leader we must **frame the situation in a way**

that allows us to see the challenge as something we can overcome, rather than impeding our progress. For me, it's workouts, for you it may differ. Find your source to draw from and grow.

The second quality is humor. When we laugh, the stress we feel melts away. Humor has been found to reduce pain by the release of endorphins, strengthen abdominal muscles, and increase immunoglobulin A, a major antibody produced by our immune system as well as two other antibodies that stay elevated for up to 12 hours that bring about healthy outcomes.

Laughter reduces cortisol and regulates growth hormone and adrenaline. Those three hormones are good short term, but when elevated for prolonged periods of time, destroy the body. Cortisol is catabolic meaning to break down large molecules to smaller molecules. It will break down muscles and other tissues as well as keep the body in a state of acidity which is poisonous when circulating in the blood for too long. Chronically elevated growth hormone can cause over growths (cancer) and enlarge organs that if any larger would restrict major functions of the body. Chronically elevated adrenaline, causes high blood pressure and strains body systems that would otherwise function with precision when only used short term.

The third quality is the attitude of never quitting. We touched on this in chapter three along with pivoting, meaning to take our energy and shift directions when things are not working so as to get to the root of the results we desire. Model leaders do the same. They see reality, they understand the consequences and then they act to the best of their ability to create the reality they want, no matter how tough it is, how hungry they are, how tired they get, they find a way. To quit has its roots in death. When people quit in business, that business will die. When people quit on the team, relationships fall apart and go no further effectively killing the potential sum of two or more people. When we quit on ourselves, our spirit decays and death isn't far away. When we adapt, when we are determined to overcome obstacles, we summon energy we didn't know we had. We become resourceful and creative like we never have before. In a way, we become more alive. This attitude coupled with humility is near unstoppable.

Same Title, Different Game

> "You never step twice in the same river."
> —Heraclitus

After training hard for many days, I'd ask my lifting coach why things weren't improving. I'd put in the work, was eating well and yet some days it seemed as if I was going backwards. I was still very new and had not understood how stress, sleep, and periods of rest affected the body, but with my coach's infinite wisdom he reminded me that just because I did well the last workout does not mean this workout will be good or that I'd be able to use the same weights. It's a new day, a new workout. Adapt. Adjust to where you are now.

Of course, we are usually close to our training weight. One day of not training won't take away years of earned progress. Our muscles are still strong and we have learned more. We just need time for our bodies and minds to heal. We must train in a different way, adapt to where we are for the moment because we have created a change in our body's state. In our relationships, professional and personal, it's the same. Every time we walk into work, when we talk to our spouse and friends, we are not entering the same building or meeting the same people.

Yes, they look similar, feel similar, and may respond in a predictable way but what I mean is, nothing remains as it is. Everything is in flux. We are aging, buildings are degrading and the ground we stand on is shifting. It just happens gradually until it appears that suddenly it has all changed. It was changing the entire time, just too slow for our conscious awareness.

This may come as a surprise to many. It may even be overwhelming for some. That could be why some people choose to not acknowledge it. That way of operating though is like the child who closes his eyes thinking that others cannot see him. Reality though, still remains. As leaders, recognizing the variability of our peers, colleagues, and the environment will allow us to prepare and stand ready for when the shift enters our conscious awareness. We are less likely to be negatively surprised and more likely to meet the needs of the people nearest us and prevent disaster by being proactive.

Study the changing seasons, figuratively and literally. Understand the forces of nature, environmentally and socially. See what remains true across domains, see what changes. When we know consciously, then come to feel these changes in the people and places we share, our ability to lead becomes more effective and our results more profound.

Meditation, Mindfulness and The Breath

Now mainstream words, mindfulness, meditation, a focus on the breath, have been around for millennia. The reason it's included here is two fold. Mindfulness creates awareness of the self and the outside world. Much of the day, as we learned in chapter 2, is run by habit patterns. We pass through the day without noticing much unless there are dramatic changes in positive or negative ways. This is how the average person lives. It's not bad but it's not good. Mindfulness cultivated in meditation is not just for a moment of peace, though it does provide that on the surface. What it does is focus attention on the non-conscious automatic process of our breathing.

Why is that important?

Because **if we can become aware of the automatic process of our breath, it creates the capacity to become aware of the automatic processes and patterns outside of ourselves.** Those processes include the dynamics of our families, our teams and business. We, in essence, can see what others are unaware of, giving us vision and with the vision to see the unrealized world, we can either use it for further growth if it is helpful or eliminate it if it is harmful.

A study done by Cornell University found, after studying 72 top executive business leaders, that self-awareness was the strongest predictor for leadership success. Because we are able to see ourselves more clearly- our strengths and weaknesses, faults and improvements, our struggles and success- we can get those around us who can compensate for our weaknesses while we work in our domain of strength and also see how those around us achieve the results they produce.

How does one meditate mindfully?

Find a quiet comfortable place to sit or lie down with closed eyes and begin. Eyes are closed to remove distraction from outside stimuli. As you progress, this technique with eyes open may be used in more chaotic situations but for now quiet and calm is best. Close your eyes, and take three deep breaths, 4 seconds drawing air in through your nose, 1 second pause, 4 seconds out through the nose again. As you get the rhythm of the in-going breath and out-going breath, you may drop the count of each breath and rather count the cycles of each in and out-going breath. In-out being one cycle.

Begin with 5 minutes. Set a timer with a low volume, soft sound like a gong to know when to stop. Feel the air enter your nostrils and travel deep to your core. It's a breath with the diaphragm. Watch it as it turns and becomes an out-going breath. That's one cycle. You may notice your mind wanders after several seconds. That's okay and natural. Mindfulness is trained. Bring your awareness back to your breath and restart your count. To become the most proficient in self-awareness requires daily practice. You will not do this well every time but will get better every time you do it. **Remember, anything worth doing is worth doing badly, until you get it right. Take your time. Stay consistent.** Work your way up to 20-30 minutes of this. As your practice improves, the awareness of yourself deepens, as well as your awareness of the outside world.

Try this for 90 days. Record each in a journal to see how you have grown and how your perspective has changed. Record how interactions have changed and what you love most about these changes.

Leaders are Deep Breathers

Stepping out of the "hard-charger" mentality is difficult for many reasons. The results we get can be rewarding to the point of being intoxicating and the momentum it creates makes us feel as if we are so close we can taste victory. Taking a moment out of the day to create a calm, grounded presence does both you and those around you a great deal of benefits. Everyone faces stress in their lives. It's inevitable. Good leaders, though, will take on stress more than the average person. When we are in a state of duress, it can cloud our thinking and make someone react, rather than respond. Deep breathing does many things but I'll point out three key elements. 1) It stimulates the vagus nerve, which releases acetylcholine, a neurotransmitter that is key for memory and muscle function, as well as put us in a parasympathetic state or calm state. 2) Breathing alkalizes the blood. It improves circulation and helps the blood clear toxins and waste products that stress produces. Substances that create an acidic environment, if left unattended for extended periods of time, will age and erode our body dramatically. (3) It's a source of life both physically and figuratively. Physically, we need oxygen to survive and create chemical reactions in our body. In India, they call the breath, life force or pranayama. Figuratively, people can be a "breath of fresh air." We not only literally breathe deeper around these people because we feel safe, we can authentically express our thoughts and ideas and be heard with an open mind.

H³ for Leading Yourself | Head, Heart and Hand

This I learned from the Monk Jay Shetty. H³ for leading yourself is:

- Head: Clarity of mind. This means knowing where you are going, your path and purpose and having a plan to get there.

- Heart: Understanding your intuition and what your heart wants. This is the root of your desires.

- Hand: This means service. Passing on what you've learned, what you know and aiding others in being the best version of themselves to live their best life.

Once you understand these three elements you may effectively lead others in and through the other three elements which are their heart, hopes and hurts.

> "Leaders have what is called the HPLP Gene,
> 'helping people live their potential.'"
> —Wintley Phipps

H³ for Leading Others | Heart, Hope, and Hurt

True leaders understand elements about their people. They involve their people's:

- Heart: What your people care about.

- Hope: What your people's ambitions and goals are.

- Hurt: What they fear and seek to avoid.

They seek to understand the people they work with along each of those three elements. They work to develop the natural faculties of the men and women on their team. This stimulates their nervous systems in a way that improves their weaknesses and adds to their strengths. Be patient with the people around you. It takes time for people to share their hearts, hopes and hurts. It's part of who they are and how they became that way. They will come to you when ready. All you have to do is lead well. Tactfully connect the dots of current knowledge, past knowledge and make accurate mental models of what could happen and needs to happen for the team to succeed. When the people on your team are taken care of, you will be taken care of.

Courage

A core element of leadership is courage. We recognize the literal stepping forward of a person to lead a group or being the first to take action amongst an opposition known as physical courage but that is only one type of courage. An important one, but other types of courage are necessary for a true leader.

These other types are:

- Moral Courage

- Daily Courage

Moral Courage

Moral courage is standing up for what you believe in, particularly in the face of those above you and maintaining loyalty to those below you. When your employer acts in a way that is against your moral code, to speak up and stand your ground is very difficult.

Nonetheless, if you are to live authentically as an individual and grow, it must be done. Not just for yourself but for the effect it has on the people around you and in your life. From the time we are learning to speak and even sometime before that, we have an intrinsic idea of what is right and what is wrong. We sense it on the face of our parents and our siblings. As we get older, our friends and co-workers.

If we let what's wrong slide, it makes that way of operating easier to perform and harder to correct the next time around. This can be summed up as: if it hurts the other person physically, emotionally, mentally or financially for self-interested reasons and does more harm to everyone and supports chaos rather than order, then it's more than likely wrong and should be stopped as soon as possible.

Will we need to let people go who after being trained and coached, mentored and guided but still don't perform? Yes.

Break up with people who lie, cheat and steal? Of course.

Will we challenge beliefs and deny people who at the moment cannot contribute financially? Yes.

The questions you have to ask yourself is:

- Is this helping a cause greater than my personal interests?

- How is this helping the greater good?

Knowing the answers to these questions will lead you to the right action and when possible, allow you to leave or step away from those who cannot honor this code. There will be those that are just rotten, evil, and murderous. In that case, they are wrong from the start and if you are confronted by this presence, lead them away or just stay clear of them. If you are unable to do that and are cornered, eliminate that presence. A group needs a centripetal force to give it unity and cohesion, a cause greater than the group. By acting for the greater good, we maintain the momentum of that force of goodness. Acting in this way may cause harm to you and that comes with the territory, but the sacrifice made will help ensure longevity among the people you are serving.

Daily Courage

Daily courage is doing the best you can with the circumstances you are currently in without complaint, whining or murmuring. It's accepting what is and making it the best of it.

This has roots in the small things of life. Getting out of bed in the morning and touching both feet to the floor. Being able to use the bathroom without assistance. Waking from class to class, driving, reading, listening to someone talk or watching the waves lap seafoam onto sun kissed sand. Some people never get to have those experiences and because of that they have no point of reference. They cannot compare. What they have is all they know. Those who have had it and lost it, sometimes without rhyme or reason have a deep understanding of the gifts of health and vitality.

A soldier who steps on an IED and loses his feet or is shot and paralyzed from the neck down now has just effectively ended his mission and now must begin finding his next one. Only now with infinitely more obstacles than before. For men like Canadian sniper Jody Mitic and special forces marine Derek Herrera that's a reality. Simple things like taking a shower, using the bathroom, going out with friends and family are now a challenge. Has it led them to become innovative and tackle problems they otherwise would have never participated in? Absolutely.

Could they have prevented it I believe they would have, but the point is these men begin everyday with courage.

That even without the basic necessities they make a way and propel themselves into environments that continue to develop them and make them more than what they were the day before. For where they lack in one place, they make up for in attitude, character and spirit and more often than not, in skill and efficiency.

My best friend, Rj Nealon has Cerebral Palsy (CP). He's taught me more about living and adventure than my most able friends. Having a stroke when he was born and having seizures from a young age, damaged the right side of his body. He's had surgeries and has been hospitalized countless times. For years he would have dozens of seizures in a day, yet he's a blue belt in Brazilian jiu jitsu, rides motocross, jet skis, and skateboards. He was even a starter on the high school football team. He's a Special Olympic swimming champion with records in Nebraska and was a better swimmer than some of the kids I swam with on the high school swim team. He's currently earning a degree from Alabama University and graduates in December of 2019 with a Sports Journalism degree. To put the icing on the cake, he's earned an internship with ESPN, a dream of his since he was a kid. Does he still have bad days? All the time. Does he get rejected or beaten by others? Yes. The reason he accomplishes what he does is he does the best he can with what he has and can laugh at himself and the situations he's in. He sees obstacles as a way to better himself and become victorious. He's writing a book about his life experiences. Check him out at Nealonsports.blog for articles and updates of current sports events and reach out for more information on his life. He's more than happy to share his wisdom.

The point I'm making is this:

Even though you've been knocked down, you're not knocked out. When the smoke clears and you can communicate, you can begin to create again. These men as well as the countless other men and women who have similar circumstances yet overcome them are exemplars of what is possible with the proper attitude, spirit and being surrounded by positive influences.

Wisdom

If it seems as if leaders get all the perks, that parents or coaches get the most benefits, remember that they, if they earned the position, lived into the experience of what it means to be a father, a mother, a leader. They toiled, suffered, sacrificed and went through the rigors of learning and failing, trial and error and have now come to you with experience and knowledge to guide you and make the "path less traveled" simpler to navigate. They want to save you time so you can do more for yourself and the community and live a quality life. Rainer Maria Rilke says this well in Letter No. 8 of what became a book called *Letters to a*

Young Poet, speaking to a Young man who has been writing Mr. Rilke for advice:

> "Don't believe that he who seeks to comfort
> you lives untroubled among the simple and
> quiet words that sometimes do you good.
> His life has much difficulty and sadness,
> and remains far behind yours. Were it oth-
> erwise, he would never have been able to
> find these words."[142]

Not everyone who gives advice is worthy of leading. Part of being a leader is knowing how to filter the information and advice received and being careful about who one goes to for advice. Those who are fit for guiding and counsel will be able to connect with you with ease. Typically they will be older individuals.

Final Words

How can you find people who are motivated to work, educated and professional in their life? Fun and loving? Excited and creative?

Answer:
Become that man. Become that woman.

Do it first.

Lead by example. Don't talk like others talk. Don't act like others act. Life will challenge you, punch you square in the mouth. All I can say is, rise up above the challenges. Train constantly so when said punch connects, you know how to strike back. The only thing you can do, even when everything around you is negative, when everything is failing... is lead yourself.

If you don't lead yourself, you will be led by someone else and the chances of them being the leader you want is slim. When you control the one thing you can control, which is yourself, you contribute to the control of others and the people you need on your team will begin to do the same. Leadership, like living and loving, has its root in you. **It begins with you.**

When you become successful for yourself, you now have the credibility to make things happen for other people, when you so choose. You know a path to the result.

The fundamentals of leadership across cultures and time have not changed. Nuances exist, and different circumstances call for different principles of action but nonetheless these principles remain true:

- Leaders lead by example.

- Only ask what you're willing to endure yourself.

- If you want to motivate, be motivated.

- If you want a commitment, commit.

Leaders are do-it-first people. They listen. They listen to those around them and to their gut. If you want to lead, get yourself right first.

Closing Question:

Where are you a leader?

Where are you a follower?

In what ways are you a rascal?

How can you lead more effectively?

Chapter 6:

Gifts and Abilities

"If you work on your gifts, they will
make room for you."[143]
—Jim Rohn

We all have gifts and abilities. Most of us have a vague idea of what they are. Some have developed their lives around them without knowing what it was that had made them successful but knew that something they were doing was just right. Those that have identified their gifts and abilities consciously though, more readily rise above the standard personal successes of vocation and family to help others around them and abroad achieve success in their lives and businesses.

To understand each of these terms better, let's describe them in more detail. What I mean by gifts are those things people do or have a natural inclination for, or what some may refer to as innateness. For example, someone growing up, being more extroverted, will more often than not be an excellent speaker and be able to build rich social networks because they are always in front of others, conversing and learning how to operate in a social environment. Usually our gifts are the things we enjoy for no other reason that it brings us happiness by performing the activity. We usually don't become aware of our gifts when we are young unless adults point it out and guide us along that path. It's not until we begin developing alongside others and our gifts align with a problem others have that we can solve, that we discover we have a gift and how great our gift can be. We call it a "gift" because it, in a way, has been bestowed upon us by our environment and the people and circumstances we were involved with.

Ability is similar. Some people have a natural ability to be athletic. Genetics are a contributing factor. People who have more muscle mass, are taller, and faster will be able to outperform people of similar skill but who are not as endowed because they can move more weight, reach farther and get to a position quicker. Similarly, the person who has a photographic memory, sharp vision, and fine motor skills would have the ability to perform surgery better than a person without those abilities yet with the same training. Something most people fail to remember though is that even though we may not be naturally good at one thing, we can through practice and commitment, improve our ability.

Now to be clear, picking out a weakness and pouring everything into it for a period of time to improve an aspect of our work is good. I wouldn't recommend trying to make your weakness a strength though.

Why?

Because it takes time away from cultivating what will truly help you excel in your life and help others. Weaknesses shouldn't be left unattended to, but shouldn't be a main focus. A good rule of thumb would be spending 80% of the time working with strengths and 20% of the time working on weaknesses, challenging yourself in a new way and discovering how it can be of use for your strengths. We are naturally pulled to our strengths or gifts and in return they vitalize us and inspire others. In short, we are to cultivate our gifts and work as close as possible along the lines of excellence with our abilities.

> "Increasing our abilities, and transforming ourselves is a way we can contribute to the world as individuals as we collectively bring those skills into our families, our leadership, our businesses and institutions and even our nation."[144]
> —Ama Marston

Unwrapping Our Gift

> "At the heart of every defense lies a wound, at the heart of every wound lies a gift, at the heart of every gift lies a portal to the source of self- the

key to our deepest love and life-meaning."[145]
—Ken Page

Gifts sound sweet, caring and positive. They may conjure images of Christmas, birthdays or special moments with a beloved. The gifts I'm talking about may feel good once acquired, but the process of receiving it is far from enjoyable.

Have you ever noticed when you get a gift that the price tag is removed or scratched out? We often forget that every gift, however small, comes at a cost. The cost is usually not monetary either. It lies in where we've been injured or wounded, physically and emotionally. They are our deepest sensitivities to life. Greg Plitt, Army Ranger and Fitness Trainer said it well in reference to training in the gym: "Every gift is wrapped in pain." Similar to building a stronger, more capable body, creating what we are gifted in will be uncomfortable for a period of time and if we are to continue to develop our gifts, we will always be in some level of discomfort.

"I need you to get comfortable with being uncomfortable."
—Eric Thomas

The challenges we face at young ages are what will stimulate our growth and create a seeking to understand and overcome the barrier set before us or break us. I say young because those are the years we are in rapid development and most sensitive to change. As mentioned in chapter 3 there are different mindsets that facilitate the path we take, but all paths contain difficulties and hardship. Only one will lead to a gift. That path is seeing the situation as a challenge to be overcome and understood.

Two questions that will reveal your gifts are:

- What hurts your heart the most?
- What fills you with joy?

Within the contrast of these two questions we find what we value.

For me personally, my emotional wounds came from not seeing my mother and when I saw her, there was a problem, a fight, something wrong. Loving her, I wanted to fix them not knowing that they were unnecessary problems she was creating and that it was her job, not mine to correct them. Instead I put the weight on myself and began to seek ways to soothe, to help cope, to heal, to understand women better, to know how happy, healthy men and women treat each other. I sought ways to become stronger physically and mentally because I didn't like being hurt and I didn't like her being hurt. Now, older, I understand more what the issue was. I have forgiven her and myself for the ways each of us behaved. What filled me with joy was having my family together. When times were good, they were good. There was a sense of unity and wholeness. Being that it was

265

short lived, I valued and embraced it much more because I wasn't sure how long those moments would last. Looking back, I still wouldn't change things. I wouldn't be who I am today without them. Could things have been better? Probably, but I use reflection now to not repeat the mistakes I did as a younger man and just as important, to help others get on a path that is constructive and conducive to positive outcomes. Through that experience I came to know at a young age that what I want more of and what I want to eliminate, begins and ends with me.

> "I am the only problem I will ever have and I am
> the solution."
> —Anonymous

Will I still need the support, love, understanding and guidance of others? Of course. It's part of the human condition. The only thing I control though, is my response. With that response I can choose to seek, to expand, to let go, to find another way that is useful and productive. There are always unexpected gifts waiting to be discovered when we understand where our gifts come from and how they are formed.

> Human nature has a weak habit of taking gifts
> for granted; in times of necessity we demand
> them as a right instead of making the effort to

obtain them ourselves.[146]
—Carl G. Jung

Don't take your gifts for granted. They may remain with us throughout our lives like statues of antiquity, but even though still here, they lack the animation and vibrancy that being alive and living has. Without cultivation, the gift itself lacks the power alone to raise one to the heights of greater achievement and higher in the scale of character.

Abilities

"Where your treasure is, there
will your heart be also."
—Matthew 6:21
King James Bible

Being where you are now, with what you have accomplished, create a list of abilities. Things you could do right now to initiate forward progress in what means most to you in this chapter of your life.

Examples:

- Walk around the block for better health
- Eat a healthy meal for lunch
- Pick two new books for this month on a topic of interest

- Begin reading those books
- Meditate for 1-5 minutes daily
- Clean one corner of your room
- Study and practice to get promoted
- Call and connect with a prospect for work
- Schedule time off for quality time with family and friends
- Set up side work for the weekend for extra cash
- Write a plan for the next 6-12 months including, work, play, and romance

Read over the list you've created and then write out five reasons that will make you unstoppable in achieving those aims. Think of your greater mission, your greater purpose and the people you love. Include them in the vision of you acting.

The point of these exercises is to bring your abilities to the front of your mind and make them more tangible by putting them in writing. That way ideas can connect and you will get an idea of how much you are capable of. Knowing you are capable of more, seeing how much you can do right now will help summon the energy to do more than you have done before. Those who don't do more, will over time, get distanced and crushed.

Music and Ability

When the right song or instruments are played in an action film or love scene, training in the gym or even just at home while cleaning, how does it make you feel? I'd imagine more energized, more capable. Music sets the tone for the moment.

In contrast, I'm sure you've heard music that clashes with the emotion or feeling that is looking to be evoked. It makes you stop in your tracks or flee the area. One of the best ways to stimulate thought, remember and create the desire for action is to play the proper music or sounds. Sounds that are harmonious are considered music. Sounds that are discordant are considered noise. When I say music I mean the beats, the sounds not so much the lyrics, though they can inspire a range of feelings as well.

Why does music inspire us the way it does and put us in a state of flow?

Music, like other harmonious things, is an outlet into flow. It's as Dr. Jordan B. Peterson says: "Music is structured patterns of being laying itself out properly in the form of sounds. It's an abstract of proper being."[147] It's what the potential of an ideal sounds like organized as sound and those sounds reflect how we feel and can stimulate us to act and think in certain patterns.

I encourage you to find an inspiring soundtrack and play it while thinking of what you are capable of and how your gifts and abilities can solidify to accomplish the goals you have written down for yourself. Let the music move you into a state of flow, witness what emotions come up, journal them. Some emotions may not be good. Witness those too, if you can bear it. It will help you grow in self-awareness.

Here's a list of the sound tracks I listen to depending on the types of thoughts and feelings I wish to evoke:

- Superman: Man of Steel (Hans Zimmer)
- The Secession Studios:Dark Piano Music
- Soundcloud Ambient Music
- Inception (Hans Zimmer)
- Interstellar (Hans Zimmer)
- Zach Hemsey Instrumentals

Closing Questions:

- What is your gift?
- How can you use your gift to serve the community?
- What abilities do you possess now, today, that will enable positive outcomes in your life?

Chapter 7:

Mastery

"One can have no smaller or greater mastery than
mastery of oneself."
—Leonardo Da Vinci

THE MIND IS very tricky. We can deceive ourselves sub-
tlety and sometimes it's chosen outright because there's less
resistance or we allow distractions to get in the way. Those
who have mastered a skill, a craft, or themselves though
are the people who despite adversity, challenge, resistance,
and unknowns, continue on the journey towards mastery,
toward excellence in a skill and their ideal self. That's all
that mastery truly is, a journey with a specific end in mind.
Mastery itself is rarely the goal but rather a by-product
of activities we love and what some would call being
obsessed with.

What one on the path of mastery will inevitably find
though, is that they never truly get to the end. It always
moves beyond our reach as we get closer to our goal. When

we reach one summit, we see the next one in the distance. There's always another level. As good as we get, there's always something we can refine, revisit, refresh, no matter how basic and fundamental. In zen there's a concept of "Shoshin", having a beginner's mind.[148] It means having an attitude of openness, eagerness, and lack of preconceptions when studying a subject, or practicing a craft, art or any activity, even at an advanced level, just as a beginner would.

There's a religious phrase that says: Those that think they know, don't know and those that think they don't know, know. This is in reference to God but I'm not here to discuss that. I do believe that the truth in this phrase is that people who think they don't need to practice, study or train because they won once or know a few things, will never really know how great they can actually become. Those who are always in search, who believe they don't know enough yet, know. What do they know? They know a key element to growth and mastery.

> "If you never say 'good enough' today, I promise you, tomorrow you will always have enough."
> —Greg Plitt

In this chapter we will cover mastery in two ways:

- Mastery of Craft
- Mastery of the Self

The Process | Mastering a Craft

The term "Process" has been made popular by Alabama football coach Nick Saben. The process defined is knowing the outcome you want, then focusing on the next step in front of you in the present moment until you reach the end result desired. Other cultures teach it differently, for instance in rock climbing, they call it staying in your "3-foot world", meaning you know where you are going -the summit- but to get there you have to know your next step which is about 3 feet to your left, right or above you. As you take the next step, you get closer to the summit. In coaching athletes, I remind them, every rep you're closer, every step you're closer, every minute you're closer so long as you keep going. Focus on the next rep, the next step and you will get there and if not, you will know where you stand and what needs work. Answers are now available.

> "There's a process to how you play the game and a process to how you prepare. The process is the price you pay for victory."[149]
> —Nick Saben

A popular cliche often said to people struggling in a pursuit or trying to rush to a result is "enjoy the journey". It's not because the journey, the process of mastering something is all that great. There's a lot of gut check moments and days that drag on. Our bodies ache and our minds may feel as if they have been lost. The reason we need to enjoy the process of achievement is because the achievement itself is so short lived, it pales in comparison to the effort and sacrifice put in to get there. Thinking in terms of climbing a mountain and reaching the summit, how long do you stay at the summit? You snap a few photos, high five and then you're done. Then the work of climbing down begins. It's another journey, it's more work. It's another reason people say "love your job" or "love the work you do." It's easier to find the messages of inner and outer growth in work that is challenging, yet rewarding than in doing work that makes no sense to you for material gain, status, or recognition. In a study on love by Dr. John Gottman, he and his team discovered that anticipation stimulates dopamine longer than the reward of climaxing with your partner.[150] **Anticipation is the reward. The reward is in the process.**

Remember, if you're climbing thinking that the peak is the ultimate, it's not. You will be no better or different if you don't learn, develop and expand as an individual on the way to getting there. It will just seem like a place to break rather than to a place to celebrate. Now, will we grow up and even as adults need to do work we don't like or want to do? Of course.

When we are young, it's a time to find what our nature is and where we are weak and where we are strong. It's a way to find what kind of people we enjoy and who we clash with. As adults, it's just a matter of getting things done because it's our responsibility and no one else will do it unless we do. As children, we at an early age are pulled to certain people, places, and ideas. We vaguely formulate what we want to become and as we grow older, we refine that image, finding ways to make that interest produce income and be useful to other people, rather than just for personal satisfaction.

> Mastery lives quietly atop a
> mountain of mistakes.[154]
> —Eric Greitens

Having fixed an image of the ideal in our mind, we find if that ideal exists or has been actualized which is what we defined in chapter 3 as a model. Then we embark on the journey. Those in history who have done any great work, either in literature, art, combat, speaking, business or health all love going through the steps and procedures of their craft. Every step, even the daunting ones, excite them and motivate them. When they achieve some new standard, or some kind of record or discovery, it's rewarding, but they were so engrossed in the work it wasn't important, finding their potential was. Once recognized and celebrated, they go back to seeking, back to the way so they can get a better handle on their craft, so they can master it. It's not until the end of a long career that they find they never could master their craft, but instead mastered themselves.

Mastery of the Self

In order to become proficient, efficient, and effective in anything will mean <u>you</u> have to become proficient, efficient, and effective. You have to become disciplined. That image in your head of someone great is not something outside you. *It is you*, just not yet. This sounds obvious right? Yet so many people miss the mark.

Why?

They don't **make discipline a major force in life.**

Many times people who get really good at something don't feel the discipline. It is masked with a milieu of feel good hormones because the activity is pleasurable to them. Nonetheless, they sacrifice their time, energy, effort, money, and sometimes relationships that are not in accord with their mission to experience and cultivate mastery. That does not mean they don't sometimes feel the pain of these things, but that they don't let these things stop them from doing what they believe to be valuable and important.

Masters in history like Japanese samurai Miyamoto Musashi and Italian polymath Leonardo Da Vinci, spent their time, day and night, working on their craft. Yet not always directly or in one way. They would study some other unrelated field for use in their main interest. Musashi would study the psychology andr the traditions of his opponents, their character and how they responded under stress so he could control their reaction and set them off balance in a fight. He was undefeated from age thirteen to the time of his death in his sixties. Losing a fight as a swordsman meant losing your life. Da Vinci began apprenticing at age fifteen. Once skilled in art as a young adult, he would use this ability in another field of interest, sketching out his work when he would dissect bodies while learning the anatomy and physiology of animals and humans. He moved into the fields of engineering, astrology and aviation, creating blueprints for machines and maps of the body that to this day are proved to be true and in use. This was how they lived every day. Seeking and creating. Every day wasn't remarkable, but it was a necessary component in developing their mastery.

Rarely do you hear of romance with another person, family, or moments of fun with friends. Not that they missed or desired these things, they just would rather work on their craft. They were engrossed with discovering what was in their environment. Being that people like them choose that path, they contributed to society new ways of thinking, training and living. They established new paradigms through their work and destroyed old paradigms by changing the way we think about the world around us, as well as ourselves.

Most people are not willing to pay that price and it's understandable. It's not necessarily healthy or rewarding at first for the one performing the tasks and is a path that is filled with copious amounts of solitude. It takes a subtle shift over a long period of time with consistent practice and it's monotonous, but **cultivating mastery of any skill, in any field requires making peace with the mundane.**

It requires that we show up again and again and again and again. Moment after moment, time after time, day after day. People want the sexy stuff, the secret teachings of masters, they always want something new and exciting. That's the ego. That's the barrier. **The small things, the simple things are the sexy things.**

Most people will never experience the peak of their potential, not because they are incapable, but because they don't stay on the path long enough for them to reap results and refine their work. As mentioned in chapter two on habits, most people are slaves to what they do, they only work hard enough to get enough and not beyond to the point of freedom. Men like Musashi and Da Vinci may seem as if they were confined and "square" from the outside, but really these men were free. They had what is known as a positive freedom.

Positive and Negative Freedom

<u>Positive Freedom or Freedom to:</u> is the ability to control and direct one's own life. Positive freedom allows a person to consciously make their own choices, create their own purpose, and shape their own life; they act of their own accord rather than being acted upon.

<u>Negative Freedom or Freedom from:</u> is freedom from external interference that prevents one from doing what

one wants, when one wants to do it. These restrictions are placed on a person by other people. The more negative freedom someone has, the less obstacles that exist between them and doing whatever it is they desire.

Think of the world you live in as a building and within this building every floor has long hallways with many doors. When we are born, all these doors are locked. We are at this time, low in both negative and positive freedom. Our parents or guardians impose a schedule on us and the rules we must live by. Our choices are constrained and our beliefs and goals come from our parents or elders. We lack self-discipline, self-mastery and we have poor impulse-control.

As we enter young adulthood, we gain more autonomy. For the first time in many people's lives, there is no one watching over their shoulder. The imposed restrictions of our guardians are gone. Here is where most people veer off the path, particularly young men, but a growing number of young women too. With no structure other than what they feel is important, they can party every night, eat what they want, hang out, have fun and hook up. Life seems to be a bowl of cherries. It's intoxicating at first because being so young their bodies are resilient, the negative consequences are delayed and the good times keep on rolling.

As we mature mentally, entering the beginning of adulthood, we realize that, though there are many opportunities in life, not all of them are of equal importance. Not everyone has this shift in mindset but those that do, go from thinking they can do what they want and life is like an "endless summer", to finding there is a finite number of days to live as they are now and begin to ask themselves the question:

> **"What do I really want to experience and create with my life in the time that I have?"**

Usually this comes after failure. Failing in classes, break ups, injury playing sports or partying, going broke or being around the wrong people and paying dearly for it or some combination of all of them. If we are wise, we learn from the failure and begin discriminating our options. We have a growing awareness of what doors we can readily walk through and which require more of us to unlock. The doors that open readily lead only to a single room with a limited view; these are our lower desires. Then there are doors that take more discipline and responsibility, but once opened, lead to a staircase, bringing us up another level with better options.

As we climb the levels of our higher desires, you may notice some of the doors have bigger, more complex locks. These locks are our internal obstacles, i.e bad habits and associations. As our awareness grows and we begin to clearly define what we desire, our awareness of the habit patterns we act out also become clearer. This allows us to more clearly see the obstacles in our path and begin working on cleaning up our act to become more like our ideal.

The top of the building is Manhood and Womanhood. Here we have high negative and positive freedom. While there are minimal amounts of external restrictions on us from work or school and other outside forces, we decide that, in order to become the person we want to be, we will have to come up with our own rules and value system and set our own limits. We make conscious decisions to willingly work on developing discipline and willpower. In this process of cultivating discipline, we learn to tame and harness the power of our lower desires to fulfill our higher ideals.

By learning to tame, harness then channel our desires, we actually become more autonomous. We're not only more free from external restrictions, we are no longer a slave to our appetites. We gain the freedom of standing in a hallway of an innumerable number of doors, and gain the ability to step through any door we choose. **Self-mastery through self-discipline is the master key that unlocks the doors to the person we want to become.**

> "Simple as it seems, it was a great discovery that
> the key of knowledge can turn both ways; that it
> can lock, as well as open, the door
> of power to the many."
> —Lowell

> "...at times he may go down to defeat, but that
> matters little. What does matter is the fact that

he is fighting for self-mastery. As long as he is
fighting, he is not whipped."[158]
—Sarett Foster

A person with freedom is connected strongly to their
purpose. They know what they must give in order to
obtain their purpose and know that they are responsible
for bringing that vision to fruition; no one but you can
make that decision. This man or woman understands that
they must sacrifice things of value and embrace the reality
of where they currently are while acting in the direction
of their purpose. They take ownership and responsibility
for their choices and results; both good and bad. Having
only a negative freedom over time leaves people restless and
dissatisfied because we need limitations to feel our being.
Living a life with unlimited freedoms is not ideal. In contrast, being in control of our responses and choices by cultivating positive freedom, and working within the limits of
our existence, we find happiness, satisfaction and peace as
our by-products and live the life we dream of.

Pragmatism and Unreality | Creating Your Ideal Life

"Imagination is a force, an energy, and the mind
moves through it. And when the mind moves
through it, the body follows."
—Osho

We all have dreams. They begin as far back as we can remember. Gathering more experience and knowledge of the world, our dreams change or become more intricate but they remain with us. One cannot be just a dreamer and obtain their desires, just as one can not be totally practical and expect to live a rich life. You must integrate both. Being on one side leads to frustration. One is an illusion, the other dry and banal, devoid of flavor. In both, we find our rhythm.

Many people who immigrated to the US in the early 1900's knew how using dreams and pragmatism worked. It's the reason so many did well and the generations that came after, in essence, flopped. They had a dream, yet knew the dark reality they were in. Thousands of miles away from home, limited funds, and little space to themselves surrounded by foreigners. They had reasons to do well. They had their ideal to pull them forward and their fear of being stuck or not surviving, pushing them forward.

Dreaming | Unreality

"... if the whole is to be vividly present to the mind, and printed like a picture, like a map, upon the brain, without fading or blurring in detail, it can only be achieved by the mental gift that we call imagination."
—Carl Von Clausewitz

This may sound like an easy task but when it comes to clarifying it, getting the dream to be defined, or titled, you may find it multi-layered and vague, otherwise you would have likely manifested it. In one sense this is good, it gives you a reason to go on a journey. It's worthy work uncovering who you want to become and where you want to go and why. In another way, it's an obstacle keeping you from living it, from experiencing it.

If you want to know more about someone, ask about their dreams. Not necessarily the kind when they were sleeping, but the ambitions they've formed and what inspires them. This is the same way we come to know ourselves, only it's more subjective. Take 30-60 minutes during the week or weekend and ask yourself these questions:

- If I could do anything without fail, what would I do?
- What topics are you pulled to learn more about? To share? To do?
- What about fulfilling this dream is important to you? What's the underlying value?
- How would failing to manifest that dream feel?
- Who is with you in this dream?
- Who are you affecting? Is it positive or negative? Think about the consequences for you and others, short and long-term.

The questions and words are just a vehicle to stimulate the emotions, feelings and actions. This is what ignites the fire for moving into the unknown and attracts you to the people, places and ideas related to your dream. Then once again, when the image and emotions are clear, you can articulate them into words to share and explain what's bubbling up inside. Remember though, this is only to get us started. It will not be enough to pay the bills, build a company, hold a position of authority or mold yourself. This is where practical thinking comes in.

Pragmatism | Practicality

William James, a prominent psychologist in the late 1800's, coined the term pragmatism. To be pragmatic, is to be practical. It's facing reality. It's doing the best you can with where you are and what you have. In other words pragmatism is based on two things:

- An inner ideal followed persistently with courage
- Outer achievement related to that ideal

The former requires a dream, an ideal or vision of a better future. Otherwise what is there to be practical with? And the latter is our marker of how well we are manifesting that dream through the steps and process of practicality.

Let's go a bit deeper on what it means to be practical. You may want to be full time in your passion, let's say it's music. You love it. But it doesn't pay the bills at the moment and you have other responsibilities that need your attention like your family or children. As much as you love it, your time will need to go where you're able to sustain yourself and others in your care. One reason why people say "you have to start young." It's much easier when you begin in youth, but most don't have the discipline then or the proper coaches so for the kids it's just as hard.

So what to do?

You **do what you can.** You make a schedule that no matter what, you can practice or work on that which is meaningful for you. Say 3 days a week, 1-2 hours after work or before work. This may require you to sacrifice a later bedtime for one that's earlier to get time alone in the mornings or a later bedtime when everyone else is asleep.

The time for this needs to be uninterrupted, focused and deliberate i.e deep practice as we discussed in chapter 2 on practice. Once you start implementing this, small rewards will start to surface. You will improve a little bit more each day leading you into outward achievement related to your ideal. This way of living gives you an aim and that's more important than getting good at your craft, though that's important. Having an aim is more important than just getting good because the aim keeps us focused over time, giving our life purpose, which means responsibility and with that responsibility comes value and meaning. As we move toward that aim, we learn what works and what doesn't work. We make corrections and as we keep stepping again and again and again towards becoming our highest ideal, we inevitably get better at our craft.

Ready, Aim, Manifest

Recall a time when you were happiest. I imagine it was a time when you had an aim, a goal and we're striving for it or you had the aim of just being present, playing a game with a friend or being in the moment with members of your family. Either way, there was an aim.

The way our brain is constructed is that we cannot experience any positive emotions unless we have an aim and we can see ourselves progressing toward that aim. The reason for this is, without a target we are left wandering. Everything is vague and there's no sense in action, no order. One thing means the same as the other. It zaps energy and kills morale. But when we have a goal, today has value. All actions, all steps have value and purpose. Some actions mean more than others of course, though when we reach a position, we see where we have come from and where we need to go next. We see the value in each step and then as we make improvements, we begin creating the thing that was once only an idea into a reality.

It's not necessarily obtaining the aim that makes us happy though. When we obtain the aim, the game ends and in order to fill our tanks again we have to create a new aim. It's similar to the life of Sisyphus. Sisyphus was the king of Corinth and known for his trickery. He cheated death twice before being sent to the underworld to be punished by rolling a stone up a large steep hill and once to the top the rock would tumble back down. Doesn't sound like much fun or like there would be any happiness found there, but author Albert Camus suggests a different perspective: to imagine Sisyphus as happy.

Why?

He accepts his punishment and the task he must complete, though the task is difficult and daunting. He's turned something wretched into something he can achieve daily. The struggle to obtain a goal, though it may be trivial and difficult, is enough to provide purpose in a world that doesn't readily provide purpose or value for us. Our parents help assign them when we are young, teachers guide our values system as we mature, but as adults we must assign values ourselves, particularly in jobs we don't like, tasks we don't enjoy and things we don't want to do. The company and the people around you all have agendas and if you don't assign a purpose or aim for yourself, the one you get will likely feel like punishment rather than fulfillment.

If you can create an aim, you know there's an end, which gives you a reason to persevere and when it ends and you're at the top, you win. Even if the rock rolls back down, you completed the task and you know how to win now so there is confidence in the next round.

> ""The struggle itself... is enough to fill a man's heart. One must imagine Sisyphus happy".[160]
> —Albert Camus

It's in the pushing of the stone or in the case of modern living, towards the result that brings fulfillment. It's who we are becoming rather than what we get. Though, **what we get, will be the result of what we become.** We are much more activated by having an aim and moving towards it than by attainment of the result, though the result is important to progression, the movement toward the aim is important to happiness. It's in the seeking that we find our peaks.

Blinding Ambitions

In an experiment done by Danial Simons and Christopher Chabris in 1999 to find how zero-sum attention affects what we see, these researchers organized two groups of people. One in white shirts and one in black shirts. Each team would pass a ball back and forth between themselves. The task of the observer was to count the number of times the ball was passed between players of the white shirts and ignore the black shirts passes. While this happens a man in a gorilla suit comes into view of the camera near the middle of the activity, beats his chest and walks off.

To much surprise, most people didn't see the man in the gorilla suit do this. They were so focused on counting the passes that they missed something so obvious and potentially dangerous entering the scene.

This means two things:

- You see what you aim at. Aim is the belief and you see what you believe to be important.
- Ambition can blind you to reality, yet it can also illuminate reality.

In setting goals and standards, be aware that if you are too wedded to a path, your ambition and the goal you set may be your demise. Gather people unwedded to your plans to offer objective views and stay vigilant to the environment you're in. Ambition is an attractive trait when disciplined and controlled. **Know when you need to step back and allow the work you have done to work for you.** In chapter 8 we will discuss more on how to do that.

System Setting | Goal Checking

When it comes to goals, standards, things we want to have or become, you often hear someone "setting" a goal. People do this often at New Years. They have this great idea, they can see what they want, they know why they want it, yet they fall short and it's not even beyond the 15th day of them embarking on the goal.

Why?

Their system was bad. They didn't have a way to keep them on track. They didn't create a plan, a set of steps to follow when interruptions and distractions reared their head and they will. They got carried away and the habit took its course. By setting up the proper system, we are setting up a way to build a new habit and a way to automate our way to our goal. We set the system, the plan, the method and then as we progress, we check how close we are to the goal. If we are not close, we adjust. If we are close, we keep going. Once obtained we create a new goal and then set another system up to achieve that goal.

Let's define what a goal is, what a system is and what they each do for us.

- What is a goal?

It's an end state we are seeking to achieve. An ambition or aim we desire.

- What does a goal do?

It sets the direction for where we place our energy. We go the direction we face.

- What is a system?

It's a set of principles or procedures according to which something is done; an organized scheme or method.

- What does a system do?

Keeps us on the path towards the goal, particularly when fatigue, distractions, interruptions and fears are present. It is our rod or staff to keep us steady.

Anddddddd it's Gone..

Success is fleeting. One moment we *are* victorious, the next moment we *were* victorious. Like goals, successes have an end state. Some are long and some are short, but they have a defined end. For the truly successful, being successful isn't the goal, excellence is. Excellence is a systematic process, it's a practice, it's continuous, there's no end to it until we die and even death is something we all have the opportunity to do well.

The goal is where we want to be, who we want to be and where we want to go. The system we set is how we get there. It's the steps, method or plan. A good way to see this is in the sports arena. The most successful coaches tell their players not to worry about the scoreboard, but rather focus on the next move and then the one after that. Looking at the scoreboard won't help you score points, whether you're winning or losing. Focusing on the next move will, though. Check the score, sure, but that's not important. As Bill Walsh says "The score will take care of itself."

- What defines a good goal?

A good goal is specific, compelling, intentional and simple.

If the end state you are describing is too complex to explain or the result too vague, you won't know when you obtain it. Keeping a goal vague is easy because it protects us from the feeling of failure while we are acting in the direction of the thing we want, but it also prevents us from knowing if we have won. We may get a glimpse of it, or feelings like it but neither are it. **Unless there are clear parameters for what constitutes a win, you don't have a goal and you won't know when you have won or not.** If it's not compelling, you won't push for it. When you set this target, everyone and their grandmother will seem to get in your way and want your attention. They will try to pull you away, mostly unconsciously, into their agenda.

Stay focused and know why this is important and why it <u>must</u> be done. Know the reason you should give your energy. It should inspire you. Once it becomes routine and you start getting results, people will back off and some will even ask how you did it and how they can join you and begin making progress in their own life. If it's not intentional, you may be happy with the result that happens but it's not a goal and it also won't bring the sense of accomplishment that comes with setting a target and then achieving it, conquering it or becoming it. Make it specific, compelling, intentional and simple.

The Value of a System

What makes a system valuable is that it builds momentum. The system creates a rhythm, a pattern like the beat of a song, with rhythm that you can dance to, even if the lyrics change. The beat creates the drive and ambition, the lyrics give it a defined or articulated meaning. Even when the meaning changes, having a system in place will allow you to achieve the goal you set for yourself. Once you get there, you may decide that what you wanted to do there is no longer meaningful. That's okay too, but you now know you're the type of person who can follow up, follow through and produce an intentional result. In turn, the process will help you produce meaning and value in other areas of your life.

Remember, **the system creates momentum. The goal is our growth.** When we get the goal we know we've grown. Check the goal to see how much you've grown. If you are not growing, check the system and adjust. Never focus on the goal, you will just be spinning in place like a looney toon, talking about it, thinking about it, dreaming about it and not acting towards it. Focus on the system, on building momentum and watch how many goals you achieve.

Flow Master | Meeting Happiness

"The search for happiness is one of the chief
sources of unhappiness."
—Eric Hoffer

I once had a friend that every time you asked them how they were, they'd always answer "alright". If someone went further and asked what they were working on or what they wanted to do with themselves, they shrug their shoulders and say "I don't know, I just want to be happy." Yet everything this person did was obviously not leading them there. They're search for happiness was leading to disappointment and poor choices.

Now, there can be many causes for that. Life, as Buddha has stated, is suffering. But as we learned before, what meaning we assign to events and circumstances and the people we surround ourselves with have a massive effect on what direction our suffering and pain takes us. What this person was failing to do most often was focus on one thing that was meaningful to them and stay disciplined to achieve a level of proficiency that would afford them instinctual action and thus move fluidly through their activities where they would eventually meet happiness. **Happiness and true rewards come from patience, practice, and discipline.**

The writer Aleksandr Solzhenitsyn, someone who witnessed and survived a war and work camps in Soviet Russia says this well when speaking about happiness in relation to relationships with others:

"One should never direct people towards happiness, because happiness too, is an idol of the market-place. One should direct them towards mutual affection. A beast gnawing at its prey can be happy too, but only human beings can feel affection for each other, and this is the highest achievement they can aspire to."

The activities we love and engage in are usually something we share together or that we do for others that will grow our bond and deepen our trust between one another. This helps us integrate ourselves with virtue as well as pull together our friends and family. Over time, it may lead to a stronger community and continue to expand so as to heal other distant places and allow happiness to descend upon them in their day to day lives and activities.

•••••

Think of an activity you absolutely love. It could be exercising, cooking, fishing, drawing, grappling, reading, writing, etc. What's it like when you're fully engaged in this activity? Fully immersed in what you are doing? Time may seem to have stopped. Hours may seem like mere moments and you may feel pleasure emanating from your body even as you struggle creating, pursuing or grappling with the thing you're looking to achieve. This experience is known as Flow, a term coined by the psychologist Mihaly Csikzentmihalyi. While focusing, a person isn't looking for happiness or pleasure, but it meets him or her along the way. They are designing it through their work and disciplines.

Flow is defined as, "the mental state of operation in which a person performing an activity is fully immersed in a feeling of energized focus, full involvement, and enjoyment in the process of the activity."

There are two prerequisites to getting into flow. You need a <u>focus on what's in front of you</u>, being involved with the objects or people around you in a way that is not overwhelming or boring, but enough that you can match the difficulty of the task at hand with your current abilities yet, be stretched just outside your comfort zone so that you have to adapt and learn but when you fail, it's minor and easily correctable so you may quickly return to the activity. The second prerequisite is <u>time</u>. It doesn't happen immediately but getting to that state happens faster the better you become at the task. This is one reason why people of high competency, experts and professionals speak of this experience more often than novices.

For example, if you're in good shape, running a mile may be a pretty easy warm up. There's not much challenge and may even feel like a nuisance at times to getting to the core part of the routine. It's also not going to take very long. Running one hundred miles, as ultra marathon runners do, is likely too challenging but would afford the time to experience flow and hone in on your body mechanics, your breathing, your thoughts and feelings and get an endorphin rush that would be pleasurable. After a mile run, a HIIT training routine with a new exercise like double unders or a slightly heavier weight for more reps for three more rounds may be the sweet spot for you. As you progress, your strength and ability to cover greater distances increases, you become more efficient and you recover faster. As you continue on your exercise journey into better health, with focused intention, you may find flow and thus create happiness because you are growing and learning and creating meaning, though it may only be meaningful to you insofar as it makes you feel confident and brings you pleasure in that portion of your day.

And one might argue saying "how is it that a child is able to achieve flow by playing? And why is it harder for an adult?"

Children experience flow more readily because their attention is directed at what they are doing. They aren't thinking of work, productivity, bills, any future, any "what-ifs". They are less inhibited possibly because their prefrontal cortex, which is undeveloped, contains less inhibitory neurons than adults and they act in the moment and as they gain a feel for the activity, sometimes messing it up or falling down, it's challenging enough that they can handle it. It's flow, but it's low level flow, which over time will not bring flow anymore because we need skills and challenges to mature and grow.

Kids are also curious. They haven't fixed ideas about events in life yet. Much of what they see is new to them too. As adults we have the ability to see things from a new perspective though. We can see with curiosity as well. Being more developed than children, we have the ability to assimilate information from many sources at once and create a new experience because of the ones we have had before, control more of our environment and experience deeper levels of flow. We must not discard all our past experiences for they have taught us some hard lessons and earned us some gnarly scars, both literally and figuratively, but we must use them as a guide to avoid the same mistakes and take a new approach. We can discern what scars are worth having and which are not.

Adults that refuse to go again, hold back and stay in a comfortable place, are afraid to fail, and lose or hurt themselves. **Those that see failure as a learning curve and a challenge to be overcome, become better at what it is they are interested in.** Over time they refine their skills and automaticity sets in, forming habit patterns and over time they can perform more and more complex tasks and create art and music, perform surgeries or fly a plane or coach a professional team with multiple elements happening around them or to them all while maintaining a focused state. They are able to direct their attention and mental powers to make ideas into reality. The results they produce outwardly, reflect inwardly by producing biochemicals of pleasure. It's a win-win. That's a high level of flow.

Do you have to become a professional athlete or a doctor or chef to experience flow? No. You do have to **be intentional about progressively getting better at what you repeatedly do and what you are interested in.** As a result, you may become known as an accredited professional but that state is for anyone willing and able to put in the time, practice and summon the intestinal fortitude when challenges arise.

Mastery and Happiness again and again come back to being a master of yourself. A monk named Jay Shetty articulates what mastery is excellently:

"To train the mind and energy to focus it on where you want it and when you want it to be. You are completely detached, and undeterred from all external ups and downs. You are able to navigate anything that seems tough, challenging, fun, exciting with the same amount of being equipoise, and balanced in equanimity, without being too excited in pleasure, or being too depressed in pain, but knowing how to navigate every situation. That is great strength and great power.

The Beginning and The End

"Don't start the day until you have it finished."
—Jim Rohn

Upon waking up our minds are operating in an alpha wave state meaning we are very impressionable. Ever notice that when you wake up feeling good, having your room in order, the next thing in place so you can just go, that you glide through the entire day. People are friendlier or don't disturb you as much and there is a sense of bliss everywhere you are present. The opposition is also true, what some people might call waking up on the wrong side of the bed. Murphy's law seems to follow you, mayhem seems to unfold before your eyes.

Why is that?

More often than not, it starts with how you begin and end your day.

After studying some of the world's great success stories and gathering information on their daily lives I've implemented some of their rituals and I'll list the ones everyone can do and that are simple, yet profound.

> "Process over Product.
> Rituals over Goals."
> —Unknown

We will start the night before so as to get a jump start on the upcoming day.

Evening/Night time Rituals:

- **Set breakfast utensils and water out in the kitchen for when you arise.** Have breakfast food out if it's not required to be refrigerated and if it is, have it where it's easy to grab.
- **Have your meals packed** for work and ready to grab in the morning.

- **Set your outfit out and in order** of how you like to dress.
- **Have a book next to your bed** so you can read before you fall asleep. I recommend success stories.
- **Have a notebook and pencil/pen ready** on the nightstand or book stand where you will write your 1-3 goals after hydrating in the morning.
- **Have a set bedtime and stick to it.** Lights out. All of them and make the room cool. 63-68°F (17°-20 C°) optimally.

Morning Rituals:

- **Wake up and don't hit the snooze button.** Get out of bed and hydrate with room temperature water. Add a squeeze of lemon for alkalinity and vitamin C. Use the bathroom if necessary.
- **Make your bed.** Pull the sheets tight, flatten the covers and square the pillow. Do this as if you were setting it for a guest. You will thank yourself when you get home and ready to sleep after work and training.
- **Dress.** Look sharp and be sharp.
- **Write your goals down.** This will set your aim for the day and provide a reason for working hard. Make them simple and clearly defined.
- **Eat a wholesome breakfast.** Not that jimmy dean shit or some gas station sandwich. Healthy

fats (avocado, olive oil, coconut oil, or ghee) and complete protein (egg, chicken, fish). If your triglycerides are high, go for a complex carbohydrate like oatmeal and some berries, add water, blend it up and go.

- **Turn on educational/motivational material on your commute.** Learn something. Find a podcast or channel that offers something useful you want to or need to know more about. Good podcasts and channels are:
  - Jocko Podcast
  - Jordan B. Peterson
  - Impact Theory
  - Healthy Theory
  - Bite-sized Philosophy
  - Cardone Zone
  - Bite-size Philosophy
  - Grant Cardone Real Estate
  - Habits of the Wealthy
  - Ben Lionel Scott
  - Chispa
  - Academy of Ideas
  - Coach Corey Wayne
  - Mulligan Brothers
  - Joe Rogan Podcast
  - WisdomTalks

Some of your commutes may be short. That's fine. Some of these channels have 5 minute clips. Something is better than nothing. Start and the way will open.

- **Keep your phone on airplane mode** unless you are making client calls or your on-call. While at work, work. If you're playing on the phone, you're practicing becoming distracted and divided. Practice focus and wholeness, even when the tasks are wretched, be there. It ends and the focus and attention you develop through this will be significant. It will reflect in everything you do particularly in your relationships and how you problem-solve.

Closing Questions:

- What do you want to master?
- What have you mastered?
- What area commands your attention and where do you excel naturally?
- What are 5 goals you will set for yourself for the next 3-12 months and what system will you set up to obtain these goals?

Chapter 8:

Sabbath

"Rest and self-care are so important. When you take time to replenish your spirit, it allows you to serve others from the overflow. You cannot serve from an empty vessel."[166]

—Eleanor Brown

In late September of 2017, I was starting to get into a smooth routine. There was steady work pulling cable, I was beginning to grasp the fundamentals of cabling and installing the hardware that goes with it. After work I would run and do a series of calisthenics, then it was time to read and take notes. All summer I was in this mode of operating and I was becoming really efficient even with little sleep, minimal meals or being fasted while still taking on the stress of work and relationships in my personal life or so I thought. I felt I had some control over my day and myself again.

I started pushing myself further and further on my training routines after work to see how much I could do and to relieve some tensions from a breakup that I had not reconciled myself with. On those days that those particularly dark feelings would wash over me, typically on the weekends when my schedule was open, I'd run, literally, outside in my neighborhood. Usually a mile and a half later, I was feeling better then I added another loop, which is 0.7 miles then another. Soon I was doing 4 or 5 miles at a time. I did this 3-4 days a week, along with gym workouts on and between those days. When that became easier, I added a 24lb vest and worked up to 4 miles in 41 minutes. I was feeling good. I noticed in the mornings though, I would wake up just beat up feeling. To describe this feeling to others I'd often say it feels as if I was "dipped in acid", which in a sense all the lactic acid I was making, wasn't too far from the truth. In short, I was over training, over working and under recovering.

Ignoring the signals and thinking I could just work through it, I made a challenging workout day. It started off with a run, then a gym workout then a pool workout. The run was to 14 miles, 100 pull ups, 100 push ups, 100 sit ups, 50 5-count flutter kicks then a swim of 5000 meters. I drank a coffee and had two water bottles the morning of September 29, 2017. I was fasted and just started running. What was I thinking? Apparently, not about performance. I got a runners high around mile three, once I came down a bit, I felt fatigued but kept going. Around mile twelve, I was forced to stop and walk from a pain in my lower back. I walked about 100 yards then started running again. I wouldn't quit. I was so close. I decided to take a different route that added 2 more miles to the run. Once done, my knees were swollen, I craved protein and choco-late -weird combinations right? I'll explain later- and was feeling spaced out. I finished the run in two hours and two minutes. Before going to the gym, I bought some liquid egg whites and chocolate coconut water. Once in the gym, I finished the liquids and went to town on pull ups. Two sets in and my bladder was full, which seemed fast for just finishing the drinks. Took a break and went to "bleed the lizard" when I looked in the urinal and saw thick red blood pouring into the bowl. No pain or stinging, just red. Not clear red like when you drink beets but dark red like when they draw blood at the doctors and put it in viles. Being so tired and withdrawn, I had no emotional reaction. My first response was "that's not good." And called several people to see what to do. Not long after talking to a gym friend I was on my way to the emergency room for blood tests and IV bags.

The results:

Rhabdomyolysis aka acute kidney failure.

I had pushed myself too far with too little preparation and paid for it in more ways than one.

I was told by the nurses that I couldn't train for 2 weeks or do anything strenuous and that I needed to slow down. Which at the time felt like being grounded but I knew they were right. After further reflection, I realized I needed to listen to my body and take time to recover. Had I listened I wouldn't have to take fourteen days off. The reason I was craving protein was because I had broken my muscle down faster than I could recover and the result was I was literally urinating it out.

The reason for the odd cravings was coconut water is said to be the closest thing to blood plasma and it has electrolytes for helping to balance fluids in the body. Chocolate has magnesium and that helps with relaxing muscle tissue and reducing stress alongside hundreds of other biochemical reactions.

I was thinking I could get by with close to nothing and perform at my best. It may work once or twice but only because the tank was full enough from being rested, fed and sufficiently loved beforehand. As we discussed in the chapters above, we don't just will a monumental feat to happen in an instant. **We build strong foundations over time, little by little, progressively, each part playing a role, no matter how small.** Each aspect must be given the proper attention and nourishment for growth. The time to will it, to push beyond a limit is not every day. Push hard, yes, exert will, yes but it shouldn't be a max out day 7 days a week, 52 weeks a year. That's a recipe for an early grave.

"It's a short hop from badass to burnout."[169]
—Brendon Bruchard

In those two weeks of time off, I was able to get full nights of sleep, make time for intimacy, enjoy warm meals with family, study without being mentally fatigued and more importantly, be fully present in each moment. I realized I wasn't going to "wither away" or "lose all my gains", that I could in fact deal with stress in ways other than physical exertion and still come away feeling accomplished and like I was making progress in developing myself.

More than a year later, I was doing some reading on masculine personas and drive and how it can get men into some places they don't need or want to be in. The passage said this:

> "It is a balance between the stubbornness to see something all the way through to failure or success, and the ruthless fluidity to abandon your plans and pivot when you know you should."

I believe this applies to both men and women because both men and women can enter a state of masculine and feminine. Gender and presence are different. And don't get me wrong, I'm proud I finished, I'm proud I performed at that kind of intensity and then, even with rhabdomyolysis, went to work and kept other aspects of my life in balance but I also know I was stubborn and didn't need to do that. It was a waste of time and money in the way I went about it. Knowing what I know now, the preparation would be much more thought out and my nutrition would be dialed in rather than a spur of the moment compilation of cardio and aerobics with some liquids to "hold me over". I was acting like a weekend warrior instead of a true warrior, a true student of the game. Make no mistake though, there is a time to push. Injury is not the time to do so, unless not pushing, leads to death. Rest so you may push. So you may drive on harder, faster, and stronger than you have ever done before.

> There is a time to be ahead and there is a time to
> be behind. There is a time to be safe and there
> is a time to be in danger. Just as you breathe in,
> breathe out.
> —Dr. Wayne Dyer

This chapter on sabbath is a reminder that rest is a necessity, despite what motivational speakers, soldiers, or wild type A people say. They say this to get you in the game but once we're in, we must learn to discern from what serves us and what's excess. At times we have to diverge from our work when our tanks are empty and find our oasis of safety and relaxation to heal and come back stronger and more resilient. Rest is where not only our bodies grow and minds are able to expand, but a time for our spirit to grow, our connection to ourselves to deepen and our connection to our loved ones as well.

I'll rest when I'm...alive

An ex-girlfriend's mother once told me, when I was a teen-ager, and refused to go to the store in the early morning with her and her daughter that I could "rest when I was dead." Moms really do know best or do they?

Many people share this mentality and usually say it in regards to something they want you to do for them or with them, or for things that are socially constructed like gath-erings, parties, outings and the like. Rarely is that phrase stated for things that matter a great deal to us personally. Activities we love and people we love energize us and when they don't engage us, that's a potential signal for rest and space from the stimulus for a moment. I believe intrinsi-cally we know how important rest is for our bodies and minds to develop. **Taking rest when we know we need to is self-discipline.** That's self development. That's a man. That's a woman. Knowing oneself and one's needs, and get-ting them met. The wise ones have done the preparations before a big test, have squared away the house and finished chores before going to the pool party, trained diligently for a competition and are well rested so when it's time to play, party or perform, they have the energy, patience and pres-entness to be with you or the task at hand as their best self.

There is Action in Inaction

Our brains have two distinct modes:

- Default mode
- Central executive mode

The term default mode, made popular by neuroscientist Matthew Lieberman in his book *Social*, is when our brain is essentially mind wandering.[167] Our thoughts are directed towards people, projecting ourselves into particular scenarios with them, how we would respond to this action or that situation, basically daydreaming. It's a key component of creativity. It happens and is facilitated by states of rest and relaxation. It is difficult to daydream when danger is lurking around the corner, literal or imaginative and if you are daydreaming at the moment danger is around, either you're bait or you're so distressed, you detach and become more of a witness rather than a participant in what's unfolding.

The term central executive mode made popular by Danial J. Levitin in his book, *The Organized Mind*, is when we are laser focused and attentive to the task we are working on.[168] As mentioned earlier in chapter 2, the average time to stay attentive to a task without fidgeting or mind wandering is approximately 52 minutes. So those that say they are working for hours and hours every day at the library, in the gym or at home are giving you the runaround. They may be in motion but not in action. We've all been there. You get tired either because the task is mundane or not of much danger and we just float on through the task not paying attention to what we are doing. Napoleon Hill calls this "drifting" and it leads to trouble. If we are lucky, which is not something to ever count on, then the task is done and no harm is done. Which is just as bad as an injury because you failed to notice it could harm you or someone else and got away with it. Usually it takes a mistake to wake us up and focus again, though if you rest and then get into action, it doesn't have to.

In contrast, while in action, we are alert, conscious, fully engaged and aware of what we are doing. We are present. That is when we are most alive and are enjoying ourselves regardless of the task we are doing. Things may get done when people are in motion, but it's more than likely half ass and probably not remembered if it is done well. When we take the proper rest between sets, either in the gym or in our tasks at home and work, we effectively allow our minds to do as they have been divinely designed to do and we perform more qualitative work. On the second floor in the Department of Laboratory Medicine at NIH there's a picture that says "Quality: the name we give to the work we do." **Everything we do, we leave our name on it. It's a symbol of who we are. Being well rested, well prepared ensures what we do and who are, are in alignment.**

The way we become well prepared is by taking time away from our work to get into a state of relaxation and ease for a short period of time. This is where our minds will bring forth ideas and solutions. Everyone's idea of this may be different but I imagine it has to do with a organized clean natural setting, family, friends or both, food, music, and sleep. All of these elements create within us well-being, harmony, and a connection to ourselves as well as the world around us. When we not only see our family but connect with them, our bodies recover faster from stress. When we eat good food our bodies can grow stronger. When we sleep deeply, our minds and body can become more resilient.

> "Tenderness and kindness are not signs of weakness and despair but manifestations of strength and resolution."
> —Kahlil Gibran

We are more likely to be kinder to those around us and more understanding too. As our bodies require food, water and oxygen to survive, hard work requires rest, relaxation and inactivity to allow us to enjoy the labors of our work and flourish.

Take or Be Taken

If you don't take the proper rest when it's the proper time, the proper rest will take you when least advantageous. Read that again. When it's time to go to bed, go to bed. Turn the phone off or on airplane mode. She can wait or he can wait and if they cannot, they don't value you or themselves. The next day is coming weather you are rested or not and it doesn't care if you feel good, look good, or bad, it's bringing all the activities, customers and opportunities to you and the only way you can perform at your best, be of service, and capitalize on the day as it unfolds is if you are in the best state of mind and body. If you are not, it will be twice as hard as it was before because you'd have less energy and less clarity. Sleeping as we discussed, is a major key. It not only heals us but helps us make better decisions by keeping our prefrontal lobes, the place of our executive functions, working optimally. We can control our impulses and desires and maintain discipline which in turn, over time will lead to freedom to go and do what we choose to do when we want to do it.

No means No!

Your mom probably told your sister this as she got older when the boys started to come into the yard and just like her, you need to know when to say "No." The word "No", though it is a negative term, can have positive effects. It's not for beginners. Why? They have no experience and to deny a chance to learn and grow is immature at best and idiotic at worst. You may hear salespeople teaching "yes, yes" or hear the rich or famous people telling others to embrace "yes". It's for those who are new. It's for those who are just starting their journey. Humans by nature and on average have a negative bias. Positive is not normal. People like things to be constant, they dislike change. That means people won't try new things or go to new places and that leads to a host of other negative associations and consequences.

People who win, people who are titled "successful" are those that are able to discern what's valuable and of utility in their journey and what's not. Saying "yes" gets you in the game, saying "no" allows you to keep playing and play for higher stakes than others so long as your "yeses" have been fruitful. With negating, you essentially maintain what you have, which when you have reached your goal or destination is key to enjoying the place you're in. It puts you in a position of power over yourself and situations because you are determining your direction rather than being pulled into another venture. Saying "No" is equivalent to pumping the brakes to make turns and come to rest and reset.

> "When you take your time, work seems less like a slog and more like play."[169]
> —Brendon Bruchard

When you know what to say "no" to, you've entered the long game. The long game means acting in ways that ensure mission success. You're not looking to get rich quick, you want to get rich for sure. You don't want to be fit for the summer or for a season, you want to be fit every season, all year, every year. You don't want flings (some would beg to differ), you want authentic love and companionship, someone you can trust until you die.

Now to be clear, if you're doing what you're doing so you alone can get ahead for whatever that means to you, you will likely fail. The only way you will sustain the levels of energy and intensity as well as take the rest you need, is when what you do is for the people in your circle, your family and teammates. You have to have something greater than you that will allow you to say "No, I'm going this way" or "No, thank you but I'm doing this." **Find your reason to do better, to be better, to rest and rejuvenate so you don't deteriorate. You're needed. You're valuable and by taking your time and resting when you've earned it, you communicate that.**

To know if you "earned it", ask yourself:

- Did I give my best?
- If I went right now again, at this task or what is being asked, could I honestly do it better or sustain my performance? Take a moment and think about it.
- If rested, how much stronger, faster, more prepared and ready could I be?

It should be obvious when you earn it. If you don't know, get an objective perspective from a credible person that is believable and resilient, someone who has gone beyond where you've been and conquered it well, not just barely made it. You should know when you earned rest and when it's needed.

Reflect in Rest

> The years teach much which the days never know.
> — Ralph Waldo Emerson

When we are resting, our mind wanders which for some can be terrifying. Embrace that. For many, it's a chance to find their unbounded creativity again. Embrace that. Here's an exercise for you and it's harder than you think not because it is strenuous but because in a culture that is always on the move, slowing down and stopping is for most, hard to fathom.

The exercise is:

Stop, sit and be still. Observe yourself and what sensations are happening inside and outside your body.

Next, take a moment and observe where you are with your eyes, then your ears, your nose, your body and if you're eating, taste.

Next, look back on how far you've come. Look at your accomplishments. Appreciate this. Let this add to your confidence and rapport you have with yourself. Remember these things before you set forth on your next adventure.

Final Words

On the sabbath day, consider your priorities and what really matters in the end. Focus on that and what you truly desire will more than likely come to fruition. Some sabbaticals are short and some are very long. Depending on the work you do, you may take as long as a year off to reflect, rest, recover and find your inner peace. In some white collar communities, for every ten years of work, they take one year off. These people read, write, sail, travel, and sleep in. They let their soul catch up to where their bodies have been running to. This may not be in the cards for you just yet, but if you learn the game of work and play, work and rest and you play those cards right, you may take all the rest you need, when you really need it.

Closing Questions:

- Where are you overreaching?
- What can be postponed?
- How can you rest more deeply?
- What will cause you to play the long-game?
- Who will you play for?
- Where do you need to say "No" in your life?
- What settings and people relax you?

Chapter 9:

Friendship

"The better part of one's life
consists of his friendships."
—Abraham Lincoln

A GREAT PHILOSOPHER was once asked "What is a friend?" To which he responded "A single soul dwelling in two bodies." Friends are the people who uplift us when our days are heavy, bring us joy, keep us on track and illuminate unforeseen possibilities in ourselves. They are part of what makes life worth living and often give value to our daily lives. Lack of friendship often leads to malice and evil doing, wroth feelings and action and even harm to innocent people.

There are friendships that last only throughout our elementary years, some through adolescents and others we may carry into old age. Others may form later in adulthood at college or in business and become just as close as ones formed in our earlier development.

Without friends, the wealthiest life, if it could be called wealthy without friends, would be very bland and lead to a dull existence. In fact, friends can be a source from which to draw inspiration, motivation and cultivate our energy to perform at our best in all arenas and be in optimal health.

"The moment a congenial friend calls, their very presence unlocks all the doors of the mind, the gates of the heart fly ajar, and every avenue to our affections open up to them. Their coming is like the sunshine in the spring; our whole nature warms and responds to their genial presence; new hope and courage are born in our thoughts; we can say things and think things impossible before. We become prolific, original; our powers seem multiplied. The faculties which, but a few minutes before, were locked tightly, are now responsive. Mechanical expression gives place to spontaneous flow. Shakespeare says:—

'He makes a July's day short as December; And with his varying childness, cures in me

Thoughts that would thick my blood.'"
—The Success Library

Meet People Where They Are

In the relationships that have the deepest meaning and the strongest connection for you, what is the common factor? Most often you meet them where they are. By this I mean there's no expectation of them needing to be more or act a certain way or to tone down their behavior—-though circumstances may suggest they should—but that you remain with them however they are manifesting themselves in the moment, from moment to moment and they do the same for you. There is a sense of inner freedom and expression with those whom we meet when this acceptance is granted us.

Now think of the times when you have looked beyond where people are and how the mismatch creates conflict. How did it turn out? Likely in a dispute. Let's be clear here. If your friend is messing up, causing chaos—-not just being daft in public—-but immoral and unethical, or being a bully, or abusing drugs and alcohol, you should challenge them. It's tough love, but it may be the necessary antidote to their demise. It may put them back on the path or at least re-illuminate it for them before they get lost in the dark.

Something to remember though:

Don't overextend yourself.

It's easy to want them to get better, more than they themselves want to improve. Allow them to do what they can and need to do themselves. People who do the things for you that you could do yourself will over time consume you. They may be unaware of what they are doing but that doesn't make the situation any better. In the case of a friend, it's also robbing them of a victory and would actually weaken them and the friendship you share.

Simply provide guidance and have positive regard for the part of them that's striving forward while at the same time sympathizing with the part of them that's not but do not consider that part of them that's falling short, an ally or a friend. Once you have assisted them, let them do the work of putting the pieces together.

Be Able to Stand Alone

Long time friends, even family members may challenge you from time to time with their actions or you may simply grow out of the activities each of you engage in.

If they ever get negatively emotional with you or choose to ignore you or attempt to fight with you, remain in the heat for a moment but don't get caught up in the drama. Misery loves company and most often they are looking for someone to frame as a target of their undoing. They may blame you. Simply and calmly listen for a moment and seek understanding. If a resolution cannot be created, thank them for the expression and walk away. Words spoken in anger are often regretted and not truly meant towards the other, but rather are an inner expression of one's own turmoil and agitation from a weakness being exposed.

We may tolerate them for a while but friendships aren't fueled by the hot coals of slander, aggression and meanness. Let them cool down; let yourself cool down and center and come back when you can communicate together. Be okay with letting the flower of friendship die if it has come to that. One of the best ways I've heard of going separate ways from a friend is a story of an outstanding soldier leaving the service to engage in their next mission outside military life. The leader in charge of this soldier tried to keep them in the ranks and was very disappointed to see them go but with understanding and best wishes said "It was a great honor to serve with you. Thank you for the experience."

They shook hands and parted ways.

Being able to go alone is a sign of maturity and confidence. Solitude helps to make clear what is in the psyche as well as organize and integrate our experiences we have shared with others and we ourselves have experienced during our day.

Only for a short time will we entertain the friend who "can't live" without us or who constantly needs attention and stimulation to feel connected and accepted. This type of friend in the beginning may make one feel good and feel as if your friendship is very special. The reality is, the friendship may be unique but the one who is always in need is an abyss you cannot fill. It is they who must fill their own reserve and find the strength to be with themselves. Remember, you're valuable too. Others whom you know and whom you don't know are ready and able to enjoy your company.

Good Friends | Bad Friends

> "He who comes from the kitchen smells of
> its smoke."
> —Lavater

Our circle of friends see us as we cannot see ourselves; with good friends of lofty and honest character, we seemed to be elevated and spurred on to become more and exert more of the divine within ourselves; with friends of a lower disposition, they demoralize and warp the manifestation of a higher ideal and the results of our association with them end up pitiful at best.

The definition of a good friend may vary in nuanced ways. I believe there remains universally true virtues that apply no matter the age, sex, creed or race. These are things such as:

- Honesty
- Respect
- Tact
- Sharing
- Sacrifice
- Love
- Positive Regard
- Listening Ears
- Comedy and Laughter

Giving of these virtues not only brings peace and joy to those receiving, they become part of who you are as a man or woman, part of the whole that is your being, your character, which will bring those virtues back to you, even after you have become those things. A wise man once said: "Who needs enemies when you have bad friends?". Likewise, having good friends may be what takes you to the next level of your success. Fortune may be made or marred by the friends one selects. Simply by being associated with a particular group, other people will tend to associate you with them even if you are not participating at the same level they are or the activities they engage in. What's more is, as if by osmosis, you may notice you begin to adopt their mannerisms, intonations, and mode of speaking. We grow like those whom we daily blend.

Be Selective

> Be courteous to all but, intimate with a few, and
> let those be well tried before you give them your
> confidence.
> —Georgia O'Keeffe

Our resources are finite and if we are to go as far as our inner ideal urges us to go, we must invest wisely with our time, energy and knowledge. That is to say, relationships, however enjoyable, have a cost. Some are worth the sacrifices and some are not. Some have an inflated tax which rather than restores well-being and is a source of renewal, depletes and drains one's morale. A prominent psychologist has said "relationships are therapeutic. If they are not, then you don't have a relationship, but something else entirely. Possibly something approximating Hell."

In essence, there needs to be a standard of acceptable levels of conduct and shared experience to build trust and promote stability of one's inner and outer states of being. Depending on the disposition of the individual, the level at which one shares their life with others will differ.

Extroverts seem to think out-loud and talk endlessly of everything that permeates their existence; introverts may come off as uninviting, cold and distant, possibly even hard to open up but don't be fooled, there is likely a deep reservoir of power and knowledge waiting to be shared by these type. People of neurotic nature may elicit your protective instincts and nurturing side and they themselves may share their insights and vulnerabilities more readily than someone who is disagreeable.

Disagreeable people, as coarse and hostile as they can be, are honest and forth putting of what's really on their mind so you can get to the center of what needs to be changed and know what direction they are headed; there's no hidden agendas. People high in openness will want to share their ideas and stirrings of the mind and more readily listen to your wild ideas as well. If any one of these is agreeable, then you may find they are very supportive of you and your goals and may even get on board with helping you achieve them. People who are conscientious, who are orderly, and share a sense of duty and implementation will want to share a common mission with you and take action on what it is you each believe in. They will have clear boundaries and high levels of discipline that make them reliable in crisis and when work needs to be done.

Learn about people and their nature, not just from books and lectures but from being around them, sharing a space momentarily with them and you will come to know more about yourself and what relationships are vital to your development as an individual and possibly your career. All personalities serve a purpose and some in our lives are of greater value than others. Find your friends and begin enjoying yourself, your work and one another.

Getting Through Obstacles | Battling Each Other to Success

The Obstacle is The Way
—Ryan Holiday

Every road worth traveling down has obstacles. In fact, they are what keep us agile and aware of our goings on in our relationships and activities. **Obstacles are what sharpen our body and mind for success.** The obstacles in our relationships can take many forms; some physical, mental, emotional, financial, spiritual, ect.

Overcoming obstacles with our partner, with members in our community and family are what strengthen our bonds and commitments to the people we care about most. Embrace them, particularly if you are a man reading this. The downside is they can also destroy the foundations on which the relationship was formed if not handled properly. In order to get through those tough moments you will want to keep a few things in mind. Below are some methods that will aid you when the tides begin to rise:

- Gratitude Journal and sharing what you're grateful for with your friend or partner.
- Stepping away for 20 minutes then coming back ready to listen first then communicate your feelings. (Box Breathe for 10 minutes then read something positive for 10 minutes)
- Remember your "Why" for being with them. Use photos, a song, or art to bring you back into a loving state.
- Exercise alone or together (BJJ or MMA in an actual gym, not the living room, Weight training or go for a run)

Two in particular that I have found most powerful are the Gratitude Journal and Exercising alone or together. The gratitude journal refocuses the thoughts and reminds us of the grander scope of the relationship instead of those few moments our friend or lover has irritated us (though it could be a sign to evaluate the relationship) and exercising is a healthy outlet that brings in endorphins and allows you to physically exert force without harming someone and instead sets the stage for a stronger body and mind. Afterwards, with the pressure released, the problems we once had before exercising, that seemed overwhelming, become clearer and we are able to think more positively.

Then this is the main part, **listen** to him or her.

Being this book is geared toward young men, this is not permission to be and act as a woman does when she expresses herself. They are different. Get to the point in about two sentences and without flamboyant gestures and dramatics. Whatever is happening, stay grounded; stay centered and use the adrenaline to focus on producing a solution. (Going to the gym and training makes this much easier to do.)

Now your expression can be done with a raised voice and shaking fist if that's what's in you or with quiet intensity. It depends on your character and context of the situation.

An example would be:

- When you said _____ and did _____ it made me feel _____.

Keep it to facts and subjective feelings. Both of which are irrefutable. Then leave the floor open for him or her to express themselves. And by no means do you need to explain why you feel this way. If they question it in a manner that's to put you on the defensive, ask them to simply accept that's what's there. If they cannot, accept that outcome and agree to disagree then move forward with understanding. Understanding doesn't mean you agree or that either of you have "won". It simply means you can relate and see their reality. That shared understanding strengthens the bond between you and your friend and at a minimum, removes ill feelings toward one another allowing for further development of your relationship or further progress toward your shared goals.

Be Tolerant of Differences

Even the most biologically similar people on the planet, twins, share some of the biggest differences. In fact one major thing we have in common is our differences and to move beyond the surface of what we know and see outside to the inner workings of individuals, we must, for some time, put aside the differences that alienate us and work together or at a minimum, actively listen.

These differences matter less when the mission or objective is critical. Competence and integrity come to the fore as trivial traits fall to the background. As much as you may not like him or her, if they can get you home safe to your family or keep you out of harm's way, you will likely work together because the stakes matter. When what we work on has little effect on one another, pettiness and prejudices usually seeps in.

In those moments that are seemingly trivial, find a reason that it matters and make it matter and you will notice three things:

- You will participate more enthusiastically and your role as leader or subordinate will cease to matter so long as the mission is being accomplished.
- The person or people you are working with attitude(s) will change and become more lively and cooperative.
- Time will feel as if it has gathered momentum and everyone will be in a state of flow.

Not many things are as easy or hard, fragile or resilient, fun and loving and dreary and sorrowful as friendships. They are an adventure of the soul and inspire outer quests to foreign lands. Keep them close. Keep in touch and life will take on a vibrancy that cannot be created in any other way. As we age, and grow nearer towards our end, having close friends and family nearby becomes of greater importance and may be the difference between one more day above ground or our first day in the grave.

Closing Questions:

- Who is your best friend?
- How did you meet?
- What about your friends are you grateful for?

- How could you be a better friend?
- What does friendship mean to you?

Chapter 10:

On Death: The Great Equalizer

"Every year you pass an anniversary unaware: The anniversary of your own death."[181]
— D. H. Lawrence

We begin here at the ending. This is the beginning of the end as the cliche goes. Not just of this book, but in many lives, in many ways there are and will be many endings. This chapter on Death is to shine some light into and onto that darkness that surrounds that grimly word. When we face what we fear, most often it disappears. It shrinks in light of our understanding of it. Then once sufficiently understood we may direct the course of that fear into something manageable and beyond that, into something that will illustrate to those around us that our force of character is sufficient to move through the catastrophe of loss and death. That will not only help others become stronger, you will become stronger as a result.

Life itself is not negative or positive. It just is. It's always in a state of flux. The world is indifferent to our existence. What colors death though, typically in black, is that one day, we will all experience a ceasing of being as we are now and we imagine it will be a dark vacuity. Maybe so. What's unique about human beings and differentiates us from other animals is that we are aware we die, that we expire. It's not a shock to know but shakes us when death visits a member in our community, our family, our circle.

This knowledge of our imminent mortality makes the moments we have now meaningful. To try to escape from it or pull the sheet over the eyes of our mortality is to deny reality and handicap ourselves. Remember, as in the beginning about contrast. Life and death need each other. They are inextricably linked. They are actually one process. Death implies life and life implies death. It's a continuum.

Knowing we have a limited time to develop skills, love our friends, our children and build something, should provide a sense of urgency and fervor in our day to day lives. This doesn't mean rush tasks, this doesn't mean call your mom now and say "I love you" though, she would probably like that and it's definitely not permission to be reckless. What it does provide us with is a responsibility. A responsibility to find what we are capable of, a responsibility to take control of our life. How much we can grow and through that growth, take care of others, will determine our level of success now and years after we have departed.

While still here in the flesh, we are responsible for living a life our mind, body and soul can soar in. This will take years of work. Years of disciplined effort. And at the end of a long life, if done right, will be worth much more than the sacrifices you made to achieve your aims because it helps others. When we do that, our work, our voice, our actions, will stand the test of time. History is full of these men and women. Not all their recorded experiences will pertain to us but because it's maintained its value over time, it reveals itself as true. Using that truth is a key to unlocking more of your true power and living more authentically with those around you. Once we have accepted the fear of death, we are free to live. We are essentially free to move beyond any limits we or others have set for us. Now to make a distinction here, this isn't permission to dye your hair blue or shave your head, get tattoos or do any other dumb shit under the term "YOLO". If that's what's really in you though, so be it.

Judgement Day

In his book, *Histories*, Herodotus tells a story of a king and a traveled statesmen scholar that illustrates what it means to live well and die well:[182]

Solon, a statesman from Sardis and lover of knowledge, travels to Athens to meet King Croesus, who shows him his vast treasuries. King Croesus asked Solon "my dear guest from Athens, we have often heard about you in Sardis: you're famous for your learning and your travels. We hear that you love knowledge and have journeyed far and wide, seeing the world. So I want to ask you whether you have ever come across anyone who's happier than everyone else?"

Believing that Solon would say that he the King was the happiest man he's met in all his travels, was shocked when Solon named an ordinary man, a father and soldier, named Tellus of Athens and then two men from another state, Cleobis and Biton who towed there mother 4.5 miles after the oxen to tow the cart failed to return from the field.

"While living in a prosperous state, Tellus had sons who were fine, upstanding men and lived to see them all have children, all of whom survived. Secondly, his death came at a time when he had good income by our standards and it was a glorious death. You see, in a battle at Eleusis between Athens and her neighbors, he stepped into the breach and made the enemy turn tail and flee; he died, but his death was splendid and the Athenians awarded him a public funeral on the spot where he fell, and greatly honored him."

As the king grew angry by not being proclaimed the happiest man in the world, Solon explains further:

> "I won't be in a position to see what you're asking me to say about you until I find out that you died well. You see, someone with vast wealth is no better off than someone

who lives from day to day, unless good fortune attends him and sees to it that, when he dies, he dies well and with all his advantages intact... it is necessary to consider the end of anything, however, and to see how it will turn out, because God often offers prosperity to men, but then destroys them utterly and completely."

Acknowledging that the king was indeed rich and had rule over the land and the many people there, he would still not say he was happy and good until he had died because the course of his life could change for better or worse before that time. Being that he had great wealth and was still chasing the title and recognition of happiness from outside, Solon realized that he was not truly content with himself or his state for the man who is truly happy doesn't seek praise or outside acknowledgement for he has what he wants and needs as he stands before you.

> "Nothing is quieter than happiness."
> —Unknown

When we receive praise and acknowledgment does it feel good? Of course it does. Especially from someone we admire or who is our leader. But the man or woman who is living the life they deem valuable doesn't seek those things.

The accomplishment and process of what they do is their reward. They get rewarded all along the way.

Solon points out that it is not wealth and fame and power that he is after but living and dying in an honorable, potentially heroic way. Only then, when one has passed away having lived well, meaning for a greater purpose that serves oneself as well as the men and women around them, can one be said to have been happy and lived well. Until then, Solon says "refrain from calling one happy and rather just call them fortunate."

> God himself, sir, does not propose to judge man
> until the end of his days.
> — Dr. Johnson

The Reservoir of Power | Time

What time is it?

It's likely you have a clock near you or your phone. Check the time. For as long as you live, those seconds, you will never get back. It doesn't matter how much money you have, how good looking you are, or where you live. Time is indifferent. We all have 1440 seconds a day or 8760 hours a year. Will resources and genetics help the quality of that time? Absolutely. But regardless, for those still here tomorrow, the clock hand at that time will look the same. It may say 2:47 pm and the sun may be shining and everything may be as you left it just the day before but the difference is, everything, including you, is one day closer to disintegration.

Time as it passes, passes through once. Once in the moment. That insignificant question - What time is it?- and the answer of many questions in an average day if treated casually and not thought of, is chalked up to be a time we may get to share again as just "time". That time that passes though, is our life. It matters. All of it. That being said, it's not all work and struggle. We also must use our time to think, rest, reflect and play, grow and bond with ourselves and others. That dichotomy, the contrast, is what makes life enjoyable.

Knowing our time is limited is reason to work hard towards our highest aim, earning the rest and relaxation needed to push beyond who we currently are. That way when the time comes where we have no more time here, there's no regret. We did the best we could. Death can be welcomed. Departing can be accepted. We know that it's the next step in our life cycle. That it's our time to go. With the work we have performed, we leave behind resources and tools for the next person, ready, able and willing to continue in the worthy struggle of living a good life.

"If I were 20 and had but ten years to live," said a great scholar and writer, I would spend the first nine years accumulating knowledge and getting ready for the 10th."
—The Success Library

This talk about death and mortality may sound depressing. Though framed differently, it's not. Not if you think of how to use your time well. It's not if you have a purpose and direction, if you have prepared well. So how does one prepare for death? How does one build a deep reservoir of power?

Find what is valuable to you _and_ will be of utility to others then study, practice, and teach it.

This will make you knowledgeable and articulate at the least but it's aim is to cultivate discipline which will make for a rich character. The development of character is the aim of this book and I believe an aim for those who want to flourish. For without the rich character, one who can withstand hurt and do hard things, that person will fall prey to the predators of the world and not just die, but be enslaved then slayed.

> He who has a settled determination to improve
> his mental condition will be a miser of minutes.[183]
> —Orison Swett Marden

The Richest Place on Earth

It's not Seattle where Bill Gates is or Nebraska where Warren Buffet resides. Some might say Dubai, or maybe Boston or California. Each one of those places contains riches as well as the place you live too. So where is the richest place on earth?

It's within *you*.

> "They shall say it's neither low here nor
> low there but behold the kingdom of God
> within you. Seek ye first the kingdom and
> all else shall be added unto you."

Let me unpack this a bit. We are a culmination of family and friends but we are separate entities. There is a consciousness unique to every individual and when it's cultivated and oriented properly, positive manifestations result. There is also no literal palace in you but rather a creative force. I believe God is the creative force within us. Our ideal self. Though we are not the divine, we are of divinity. Though we are mortal, we, in our infinite ability to create, are able to construct families and homes, school houses and businesses, communities and centers that survive generations after we've passed away. That's only possible by getting groups of people together that have each taken the time to work on themselves and develop into an individual worthy of such achievements.

The creative force is part of what makes a strong, rich character. There are types of creativity, some being very basic and broad, and some very niche. Being human, we came from the creative act of sex. That's our beginning. As we grow up, we find more ways to express our creativity in our family by cooking, writing, playing music, dancing, or building. Then we find an interest and work at developing it. We see errors and attempt to correct them. Something may come of it. Sometimes it doesn't. Nonetheless we are looking for ways to express, moment to moment, how we feel and perceive the world. That is one of the sources of our wealth and the keys to a wealthy life.

So as you walk your path to finding the best version of yourself or just seeking to make the place your in better, remember before money gets involved, before other people give you a hand, before your family or spouse supports your decisions, it's up to you. You will need other people most definitely but unless you begin, until you're fully committed, providence will not move to help you. The act of creating the life and environment you deem valuable will not start out as you imagine. People will fight you, and you will encounter all the things you don't want to encounter first. Once you make it past the initial hardship, it doesn't get easier but you get better.

> Don't wish it was easier; wish you were better.
> Don't wish for less problems; wish for more
> skills. Don't wish for less challenges; wish for
> more wisdom.
> —Jim Rohn

As you get better, refine skills and confidence in the actions you are taking, despite hardship, life will become more meaningful. Though the grim reaper stands in a shadow not far away, sickle in hand, patiently waiting, us creating and living, loving and learning will over time make our departure and that of others before our time, easier to bear because we have left them with more than just a few laughs and smiles but meaningful engagement, products of utility and a reason to carry on though our burdens are heavy.

Eulogy

> "While I thought I was learning how to live, I
> have been learning how to die."
> — Leonardo Da Vinci

Think about this for a moment. Your eulogy. What are the people you know going to say on the day of your funeral? What are your friends and family and loved ones going to say on your behalf of the life you lived with them? Will they mention how much money you saved? How big your house was or how nice your cars were? Probably not. What will last in their memories and what they will continue to talk about is your character, or they will talk about what you stood for and how you made them feel. They're going to talk about what is still alive here in other people, what has been enshrined in every breast, inscribed in every heart, *their* heart. That is your legacy. Today in our actions we are building that. However small, or insignificant things might seem with people, a moment of silence shared, the way you greet somebody upon meeting, your follow through on your word. They are written between the lines of your eulogy. In a moment by moment awareness and conscientiousness of the small things in your relationships, your work, and the gym, time with friends and family, you can guarantee the day of your death will speak volumes. That's everlasting life. The legacy. In doing the small things well consistently over time, your eulogy will speak volumes even though you won't be there to hear it.

Many people go about their day thinking that more is coming, that things will get better and they will for a short period of time but there will be an end to all of that. How are you preparing for the end of a relationship, the end of a career? No matter how great they are. It ends. We will have great highs, great peaks, great love, sweet embraces and hushed awakenings but those too end. We don't get them for eternity. In a way that makes them valuable. Yes, it is cliché to say "oh hug your friends and be merry and be in the moment" but that's what's real. You may not see them again, shake their hand, hug them, kiss their lips again. **There is a last time in one form for everything.**

"Chattering finch and water fly are not merrier than I, here among the flowers I lie, laughing everlastingly.

No..I may not tell the best but surely friends
I might have guessed, death was but the good
king's jest, it was hid so carefully."
— C.K Chesterton

A Way Through | Resilience

This an excerpt from the Bhagavad Gita:

"Wise men do not grieve for the dead nor for the living. Never was there a time when I was not. Never will there be a time when we will cease to be. As the soul passes through this body from childhood, youth and age, even so it's taking of another body. The Sage is not perplexed by this. Heat and cold, pleasure and pain come and go and do not last forever. These learn to endure.

The man who is not troubled by these oh chief of men who remains the same in pain and pleasure, who is wise, is making himself fit for eternal life. For the nonexistent there is no coming to be; for the existent there is no ceasing to be. "[186]

This excerpt uses the living tangible discomforts, pain and pleasure of our environment to relate them to the much more profound experience of death. Nothing compares in depth and scope as the real thing. We can only prepare so much and train to handle stressors. I believe this excerpt to mean by exposing ourselves to the uncontrollable discomforts of life as well as its intense pleasures, be it tough workouts, cold water, hot summer days, the willingness to be rejected, accepting the love of an intimate partner, we are in essence filling up our minds and bodies with the experiences needed to die fulfilled and the understanding of the transience of experiences combined with the knowing that **what we do echoes long after what we did and who**

we did it with has ceased to be. It is an indifference to the state of being alive or dying but simultaneously embracing where we are no matter the circumstances and making the most of it.

Beyond the painful part of carving out a life, there are times where we can enjoy the simple pleasures around us even in the knowing of an end or when we simply find ourselves in a difficult time. There is beauty to be found in every season.

> "The heart knows not its own depth until the
> hour of separation."
> —Kahlil Gibran

The poet Louise Ayres Garnett wrote a poem that illustrates this, combining the beauty of life's simple pleasures and deep complexities as well as a reminder that our life is tethered to death:

The Prodigal

God has such a splendid way
Of launching his unchallenged yea:

Of giving spherey grapes their sheen;
Of painting trees and grasses green;

Of sharing April rains that we

May wash us in simplicity;
Of swinging little smiling moons
Beyond the reach of noisy noons;

Of storing in the honeybee
The whole of life's epitome.

God has such a splendid way
Of tempting beauty out of clay,

And from the scattered dust that sleep
Summoning men who laugh and weep,

And by and by of letting death
Draw into space our thread of breath.

You may or may not believe in God or anything divine but a logic that you are here and one day you won't be. I don't include the poems or excerpts from others that mention God or higher powers to sway you towards believing in a faith or any such thing. It just so happens that this topic has religious and spiritual connotations. What I do want to bring your attention to is as serious as life and death are, beauty is contained in each. Each can be experienced in a way that's inspiring and meaningful. It's not all black and solemn, though it may be on the surface. It will take time and practice though to see this new perspective.

Closing Time | You Don't Have To Go Home, But You Can't Stay Here

Alan Seegar, an American Poet, serving in the French Foreign Legion, fought and died in World War I during the Battle of the Somme wrote a poem which I believe to capture more than just the friction of war and it's end but the friction, challenges and duty we have in moving towards our own ends.

I Have a Rendezvous With Death[190]
By: Alan Seegar

I have a rendezvous with Death
At some disputed barricade,
When Spring comes back with rustling shade
And apple-blossoms fill the air—
I have a rendezvous with Death
When Spring brings back blue days and fair.

It may be he shall take my hand
And lead me into his dark land
And close my eyes and quench my breath—
It may be I shall pass him still.

I have a rendezvous with Death
On some scarred slope of battered hill,
When Spring comes round again this year
And the first meadow-flowers appear.

God knows 'twere better to be deep
Pillowed in silk and scented down,
Where Love throbs out in blissful sleep,
Pulse nigh to pulse, and breath to breath,
Where hushed awakenings are dear...

But I have a rendezvous with Death
At midnight in some flaming town,
When Spring trips north again this year,
And I to my pledged word am true,
I shall not fail that rendezvous.

·····

Though not all of us are soldiers or will experience immediate life or death decisions regularly, we will all have a time
when life will get challenging and we will have to face problems and look a "dragon" in its eyes. One of those dragons
is death and though we will not win, we can defeat death
by living today and everyday with purpose, bearing responsibility for our well-being and that of our family and community, entering every space with the intent to make things
better and actually leaving every place a little better than we

found it. We can listen and be present in the good times but more importantly, in times of crisis and despair. In the process of becoming that man or woman who can be a pillar in their family and community, we set up an abundant eternal life through those hearts and minds we still live in.

You reading this, you have your start date prepped for etching into your headstone just as I do. It was the day we were born. The end for most of us is unknown. How we live in the time between then, our dash, is up to us. We honor those fallen, those passed, those present and inspire those to come in that dash. Make it count. Don't waste time. Say tactfully what needs to be said. Go and do what you need to do now so you may do what you really want to later for as long as you can. As stated in the beginning, this isn't for the "YOLO" mindsets, this isn't permission to be reckless, rather it's an incentive to be disciplined and centered. It's the realization that time is limited and it's best spent in ways we enjoy, though getting to the point of enjoyment may be arduous. Learning and loving are a couple of those ways, particularly with those people you find most enjoyable and evoke the best from you.

Get with these people, practice and participate in your passion and search for it if you haven't found it yet. Time is ticking. You have to stay until you go. Now, get after it.

Closing Question:

- How are you living your dash?

- What do you want to accomplish before your time is up?
- What do you want to leave your mark on?
- How can you leave where you are better than you found it?

My Set of Keys

> "Hormines permulti viri per pauci —
> Human creatures are very plentiful,
> but men are very scarce."
> —Herodotus

What A Man Is

In **Brandon Bruchards** book *High Performance Habits* there was an exercise in one of the chapters that asked you to write a letter to your younger self on what you could do to improve future circumstances. It asked questions like "what advice would you give them? What would you tell them to look out for? How could you be a better version of yourself?" After this exercise I was reading what I wrote closer and realized that it still applied to now.

An idea came to mind and I began writing what became a list of character traits that embody what great men of history, people I personally admire have or have emulated and ways of being that have been successful for me. It became known as "What A Man Is." Cornelius Nepos, a Roman Emperor once said "We measure great men by their character, not by their success." **It's how a person lives and works, loves and fights that defines their success.** Though big bank accounts and quality items may reflect that someone has performed well, it's not what makes them truly valuable. It's their behavior towards themselves and others and their attention and ability to direct that behavior towards abundance for more than self pleasurable experiences that makes them successful.

Here's what I believe makes a Man:

- He who keeps his word; lives with integrity.
- He who speaks the truth; lives honestly.
- He respects his body and mind as well as women and children.
- He is healthy, generous, kind and understanding.
- He is patient, calm, confident and in control of his body and emotions.
- He listens, asks questions and makes eye contact. He is curious.
- He takes calculated risks.
- He studies hard, loves deeply and sleeps soundly.
- His only competition is himself.
- He has his financial house in order.
- He places family first. He has faith in a higher power.

- He lives in line with his purpose.
- When he fails, he learns, and grows and helps others to do the same.
- He trains and prepares for the mission at hand every day.
- He feels fear but acts anyway.
- He faces the direction he seeks to go.
- He treats triumph and defeat the same, as lessons learned; he is consistent.
- He thinks with the end in mind. His actions are deliberate, his actions are decisive.
- He speaks with clarity, he can speak with everyone; he is articulate.
- His mind is his greatest asset.
- He is aware of his surroundings, aware of his enemies, and aware of himself.
- When he makes mistakes, he admits it and corrects them. He is his most demanding critic.
- He does not complain, he takes action.
- His actions speak louder than words.
- His eyes are clear and steady.
- He does what is right, not convenient.
- In the home he does what is loving. In the field he does what is respectable.
- He speaks with his body, eyes, face, and spirit; he is passionate.
- He seeks to understand before being understood; he listens.

- When a target is set, a goal determined, he stays committed to achieve it.
- He reaches the targets he sets; he is competent.
- He sees the inherent beauty in all things and finds the silver lining in all circumstances.
- He does not get tired by waiting; he is patient, persistent, and positive in all circumstances, no matter what.
- His word is his bond; he backs his words with action.
- He knows he is not the last nor the first person to do something great and knows he can learn from everyone and all things; he is humble.
- He lets go of past events that no longer serve him, emotions that do not better him, others or the situation; he is forgiving.
- He is aware of his mortality, but knows his spirit is immortal. He acts with urgency.

"It is not what one's acquaintances says about him, not what he himself thinks he is, but what he is— his character—that tells."
—Unknown

Ways To Be The Best You

The French have a saying that a man's character is like his shadow, which sometimes follows and sometimes precedes him and is occasionally longer, occasionally shorter, than he is. So long as the man is aware of this, he may not lose sight of what truly matters and who is important in his life.

Before we go on to the next list I found a story in a book called The Success Library that illustrates how some people try to veneer their being and make it more than what it seems without realizing we see what they are doing and what they really are:

"A little boy, standing on the scale, anxious to out-weigh his friend, held his breath and puffed out his cheeks, swelling himself like a little frog. The friend being the wiser boy says aloud 'oh that will do you no good! You can only weigh what you are.' One may impose upon another's judgement what they wish others to see but you cannot deceive yourself of who you truly are."

- Talk straight. Tell it how it is.
- Be kind. Be respectful to everyone.
- Speak with precision. When you speak, keep it simple. Keep it brief. Use big words only when simple words won't illustrate for the audience your ideas.
- Ask. Ask for what you want. Believe you can get what you want like a child.

- Handle objections as complaints until proven otherwise.

- Hear the message behind the words. Read their body language. Hear their tone.

- Listen. Listen genuinely with your eyes and your ears.

- Stay curious. Seeking new knowledge. New people to learn from.

- Experiment and learn to fail forward and fail fast. Use the experience for later challenges.

- Challenge others in a way that will help them grow stronger and better. Keep those around you up at their potential and they will do the same for you. If they don't, move on.

- Rest. Rest your mind and rest your body. Eat well. Sleep well. Love deeply.

- Work harder than you did the day before. The year before. Not always in the same way but always doing more, making progress toward your highest ideal. Nothing is more important than your progression forward.

- Outwork those around you. Use your mind and body together. Don't let those around you try to lure you into thinking they want you to rest. Take advice from believable people. You rest when you need it.

- Do not give freely to everyone. Be selective with your time, energy and knowledge. Be selective with your money. Not everyone deserves it.

- Believe. Believe in yourself because no one else has to or should. It's up to you first.

- Accept what is as you find a solution. Don't try to change people or circumstances. Accept where you are. It's only for a moment. Don't prematurely judge the moment. Let the situation unfold a bit. Life will happen again as you are happening to it. Take proactive steps to better the situation.

- Change what you can. That's your mind, your routine, your habits, your body, your finances, your life as you speak it, breathe it, walk it, own it.

- Take ownership of your environment wherever you are. It will provide you with purpose.

- Stay fit. Keep your heart and mind healthy. Train them and discipline them daily. Breathe and focus.

- Train your muscles to carry heavy loads and withstand volumes of repetitions. It will take you far and make you better able to lead.

- Do not follow the crowd. Go your own way. Find peace in solitude and start your own tribe. Only follow the rules or others when it makes sense and to establish a higher order of peace.

- Have gratitude for your life and where you are, as well as how many things you've achieved up until now.

- Count your blessings and count on your blessings. Good things are on the way.
- Raise your standards. Set the bar higher every year. Small steps done well. Never go backwards or sideways. Go up! Go up! Go up! But remember, success is a squiggle, it's never linear.
- Be wise with money. Buy what you need, invest in what makes you healthier, stronger, richer, more knowledgeable and will help produce more income.
- When you do something, give it your undivided attention. When speaking to someone give them your undivided attention. No matter who you're speaking with. Child, man or woman. No matter their title. Be with who is in front of you, finish speaking with them and honor them and their presence.
- Give advice based on what you have done and don't assume that other people want your advice or need your advice. Just listen. They likely know what to do, they just want to be heard and understood.
- Treat praise and criticism the same, with gratitude and thanks. They're just words. Evaluate the context of the situation and the person giving the praise or criticism before assigning meaning to it.

Thank you for your time, attention and investment in this book. I suggest you read this book 10-15 times or more until the ideas that are most useful to you have become embedded in the way you live and part of your being. May your days be filled with purpose, meaning, adventure, love, prosperity, worthy challenges, friends and family.

References

Chapter 1 | Story: A Quest

1. Pullein, Carl. "How To Define, And Achieve, Your Own Successful Life." Medium. June 14, 2017. Accessed November 05, 2021. https://carl-pullein.medium.com/how-to-define-and-achieve-your-own-successful-life-f9458e3192a1. "Success is a few simple disciplines practiced everyday and failure is a few errors in judgement repeated every day."

2. Chödrön, Pema. When Things Fall Apart: Heart Advice for Difficult Times. Thorsons Classics, 2017, 81. "Need to know"

3. Katrina Connect, and Connect Me. ""Nothing Ever Goes Away until It Has Taught Us What We Need to Know."-Pema Chodron." Karma Yoga Center. June 04, 2014. Accessed November 05, 2021. https://www.karmayogacenter.com/nothing-ever-goes-away-taught-us-need-know-pema-chodron/.

4. Holt, Michael, "The True Revolutionary: A Call to Arms by Michael Holt - Article from Sacred." Sacred - Talks, Workshops & Community, Michael Holt , 15 Oct. 2018, http://wearesacred.org/the-true-revolutionary-a-call-to-arms/.

5.   Greitens, Eric. *Resilience: Hard-won Wisdom for Living a Better Life*. Boston: Mariner Books / Houghton Mifflin Harcourt, 2016. Story ed., Letter 21, Letter 7.

6.   Peterson, Jordan B. "2015 Personality Lecture 04: Heroic & Shamanic Initiations II: Mircea Eliade." YouTube. January 15, 2015. Accessed November 05, 2021. https://www.youtube.com/watch?v=UFAyBEKKIBE.

7.   "University of Southern California." About USC, http://about.usc.edu/history/commencement/2009-address/. Arnold Schwarzenegger: " Who do you want to be? Not what, but who?"

8.   Frankl, Viktor E. *Man's Search for Meaning: A Young Adult Edition*. Boston, MA: Beacon Press Books, 2017. "the first time."

9.   Campbell, Joseph. The Hero with a Thousand Faces. Mumbai, India Yogi Impressions, 2017.

10. Sarett, Lew, Alma Johnson Sarett, and William Trufant Foster. *Basic Principles of Speech*. Boston: Houghton Mifflin, 1966.

11. Ekman, Paul. Emotions Revealed: Recognizing Faces and Feelings to Improve Communication and Emotional Life. Pg. 92. St. Martin's Griffin, 2007.

12. "40 Motivational CT Fletcher Quotes To Inspire You To Achieve The Impossible." Spongecoach, 12 Aug. 2018, www.spongecoach.

com/40-motivational-ct-fletcher-quotes-to-inspire-you-to-achieve-the-impossible/. "Get it done."

13. "Lun Yu – The Analects of Confucius." The Analects of Confucius - Lun Yu XV. 24. (415). Accessed November 05, 2021. http://wengu.tartarie.com/wg/wengu.php?l=Lunyu&no=415. "perhaps the word 'empathy'".

14. Plato. "Plato, Phaedrus." Henry George Liddell, Robert Scott, A Greek-English Lexicon, A*a*, www.perseus.tufts.edu/hopper/text?doc=urn:cts:greekLit:tlg0059.tlg012.perseus-eng1. 245a-257a

15. Gandhi, and Louis Fischer. *The Essential Gandhi: An Anthology of His Writings on His Life, Work and Ideas*. New York: Vintage Books, 2002, 210. "which can move the world".

16. Strauss, Robert L. "A Remedy for Dealing with Anxiety and Depression - Mind And Body - Utne Reader." Utne, www.utne.com/mind-and-body/dealing-with-anxiety-and-depression-zm0z14jfzwil.

17. UCL. "How Long Does It Take to Form a Habit?" God and Goddesses in Ancient Egypt: Creation, University College London, Gower Street, London, WC1E 6BT, UK, 15 Nov. 2018, www.ucl.ac.uk/news/2009/aug/how-long-does-it-take-form-habit.

18. Bilyeu, Tom, and John Assaraf. "How to Upgrade Your Mindset in 46 Minutes | John Assaraf on

Impact Theory." YouTube, YouTube, 8 Jan. 2019, https://youtu.be/UMmOQCf98-k

19. Garson, and Warren Buffett. "The Chains of Habit Are Too Light To Be Felt Until They Are Too Heavy To Be Broken." Quote Investigator, Quote Investigator, quoteinvestigator.com/2013/07/13/chains-of-habit/. "to be broken."

20. Bunch, Bob. "Jim Rohn - The Law of Sowing and Reaping." YouTube, YouTube, 18 June 2013, www.youtube.com/watch?v=xvI4djYSv0E.

Chapter 2 | Finding Excellence: Habits, Practice, Philosophy and Love

21. "Dictionary by Merriam-Webster: America's Most-Trusted Online Dictionary." Merriam-Webster, Merriam-Webster, www.merriam-webster.com/. Habits, Practice, Philosophy, Love

22. Johnson, Samuel, and Robert Lyman. "The Visions of Theodore." Elements of the Gothic Novel, www.virtualsalt.com/lit/theodore.htm.

23. Clear, James. "How to Build Better Habits in 4 Simple Steps." In *Atomic Habits: An Easy Proven Way to Build Good Habits and Break Bad Ones*, 43-55. New York: Avery, 2018.

24. Wood, Wendy. Research Gate , 2006, 2-19, www.researchgate.net/publication/315552294_Habits_Across_the_Lifespan.

25. Anderson, John R. Acquisition of Cognitive Skill. Dept. of Psychology, Carnegie-Mellon University, 1981. "Habits reduce cognitive load."

26. Nestler, Eric J., et al. Molecular Neuropharmacology: a Foundation for Clinical Neuroscience. McGraw-Hill Education, 2015. Chapter 1, 18-35. Chapter 3, 57-62, Chapter 9,227-31, Chapter 13, 304-10, Chapter 14, 326-37.

27. Williams, Ryan T. "How Science Is Unlocking the Secrets of Addiction." National Geographic, National Geographic, 22 Aug. 2017, www.nationalgeographic.com/magazine/2017/09/the-addicted-brain/. Ventral Tegmental Area (VTA)

28. Ghez C, Fahn S: The cerebellum, in Principles of Neural Science, 2nd edition, edited by Kandel ER, Schwartz JH. New York, Elsevier, 1985, 502–22 Google Scholar.

29. Slater, Matt. "Olympics Cycling: Marginal Gains Underpin Team GB Dominance - BBC Sport." BBC News, BBC, www.bbc.com/sport/olympics/19174302. "The whole principle came from the idea."

30. Clear, James. "This Coach Improved Every Tiny Thing by 1 Percent and Here's What Happened." *James Clear*, 4 Feb. 2020, https://jamesclear.com/marginal-gains.

31. Marden, Orison Swett, and G. R. Devitt. Success Library. Success Co., 1901. "Has taken possession of him.", 4248

32. Nestler, Eric J., et al. Molecular Neuropharmacology: a Foundation for Clinical Neuroscience. McGraw-Hill Education, 2015. Chapter 1, part 2.

33. David G. Psychology 4th Edition.New York:Worth Publishers Inc,1995: 43."200 or more miles per hour."

34. Sciences, Mark Wheeler/UCLA Health."In Memoriam: Dr. George Bartzokis, Neuroscientist Who Developed the 'Myelin Model' of Brain Disease." UCLA Newsroom, 10 Sept. 2014, In memoriam: Dr. George Bartzokis, neuroscientist who developed the 'myelin model' of brain disease | UCLA

35. Sanborn, Mark. The Potential Principle: a Proven System for Closing the Gap between How Good You Are and How Good You Could Be. Thomas Nelson, an Imprint of Thomas Nelson, 2017."If I don't practice one day, I know it; two days, the critics know it; three days, the public knows it."

36. Duong, Linda. Time Management Tips. University of Toronto, www.utm.utoronto.ca/asc/sites/ files/asc/public/shared/pdf/tip_sheets_study/ TimeManagement_QR_Tips_v3.pdf.

37. Ericsson, K. Anders. "Deliberate Practice and Acquisition of Expert Performance: A General Overview." American Psychological Association, vol. 100, no. 3, ser. 363-496, 1993, pp. 366–377. 363-496, doi:0033-295x/93.

38. Peterson, Jordan B. 2016 Lecture 14 Maps of Meaning: Final. YouTube, 11 Apr. 2016, http://youtu.be/AdAdf4watJQ. 27:33-28:30

39. "A Method Without Secrets." About the Violin, www.theviolinsite.com/violin_mastery/leopold_auer.html.

     "Leopold Auer was once asked"

40. "How Crossword Puzzles May Keep Alzheimer's Away." Fisher Center for Alzheimer's Research Foundation, 12 Nov. 2014, www.alzinfo.org/articles/crossword-puzzles-alzheimers/.

41. Pillai, Jagan A., et al. "Association of Crossword Puzzle Participation with Memory Decline in Persons Who Develop Dementia." Www.ncbi.nlm.nih.gov, 17 Nov. 2011, www.ncbi.nlm.nih.gov/pmc/articles/PMC3885259/.

42. Aserinsky, E., and N. Kleitman. "Regularly Occurring Periods of Eye Motility, and Concomitant Phenomena, During Sleep." Science, vol. 118, no. 3062, 1953, pp. 273–274., doi:10.1126/science.118.3062.273.

43. "Brain Basics: Understanding Sleep." National Institute of Neurological Disorders and Stroke, U.S. Department of Health and Human Services, www.ninds.nih.gov/Disorders/Patient-Caregiver-Education/Understanding-Sleep#2.

44.   Tochikubo, O, et al. "Effects of Insufficient
      Sleep on Blood Pressure Monitored by a New
      Multibiomedical Recorder." Current Neurology
      and Neuroscience Reports., U.S. National Library
      of Medicine, June 1996, www.ncbi.nlm.nih.gov/
      pubmed/8641742/.

45.   Van Cauter, Eve, and Kristen L. Knutson. "Sleep
      and the Epidemic of Obesity in Children and
      Adults." www.ncbi.nlm.nih.gov, European Journal
      of Endocrinology, Dec. 2008, www.ncbi.nlm.nih.
      gov/pmc/articles/PMC2755992/.

      Van, E, and L Plat. "Physiology of Growth
      Hormone Secretion during Sleep." Current
      Neurology and Neuroscience Reports., U.S.
      National Library of Medicine, May 1996, www.
      ncbi.nlm.nih.gov/pubmed/8627466/.

46.   Leproult, Rachel, and Eve Van Cauter. "Effect of 1
      Week of Sleep Restriction on Testosterone..." Www.
      ncbi.nlm.nih.gov, Journal of American Medical
      Association , 1 June 2011, www.ncbi.nlm.nih.
      gov/m/pubmed/21632481/#fft.

47.   "Dr. Matthew Walker on Sleep for Enhancing
      Learning, Creativity, Immunity, and Glymphatic
      System." YouTube, 28 Feb. 2019,http:// youtu.be/
      bEbtf7uS6P8. At 1:16:50

48.   Penev, Palman. "Sleep Loss Limits Fat Loss."
      UChicago Medicine - At The Forefront, UChicago
      Medicine, 3 Oct. 2010, www.uchicagomedicine.
      org/forefront/news/2010/october/sleep-loss-
      limits-fat-loss. 5.3 pounds of fat-free mass.

49. Liu, Mei-Mei, et al. Www.ncbi.nlm.nih.gov, Medical Science Monitor: International Medical Journal of Experimental and Clinical Research, 16 Apr. 2017, www.ncbi.nlm.nih.gov/pmc/articles/PMC5402839/#!po=75.0000.

50. Walker, Matthew P. Why We Sleep: Unlocking the Power of Sleep and Dreams. Scribner, an Imprint of Simon & Schuster, Inc., 2018. Pg 49, 101, 124-128, 161, 145

51. Bergeron, Michael F, et al. "International Olympic Committee Consensus Statement on Youth Athletic Development." British Journal of Sports Medicine, British Association of Sport and Exercise Medicine, 1 July 2015, bjsm.bmj.com/content/49/13/843.

52. Hadot, Pierre, and Michael Chase. What Is Ancient Philosophy? Belknap Press of Harvard Univ. Press, 2004. Pg. 38 "opportunity to do philosophy." 11, 12, 14, 16.

53. "Plato, Apology." Henry George Liddell, Robert Scott, A Greek-English Lexicon, Aa, www.perseus.tufts.edu/hopper/text?doc=plat. apol. 38a. 38a. "the unexamined life is not worth living."

54. Rilke, Rainer Maria. Letters to a Young Poet. Volume One, 1892-1910 Volume Two, 1910-1926, W. W Norton and Company Inc. Pg. 36. "A distant day into the answer."

55. Voss, Christopher. "An FBI Negotiator's Secret to Winning Any Exchange | Inc." YouTube, YouTube,

7 Jan. 2019, http://youtu.be/llctqNJr2IU. "improves performance by 31%."

56. Ridley, Matt. The Red Queen: Sex and the Evolution of Human Nature. Perennial, 2003. Chapter 5: The Peacock's Tail. Pg. 129

57. Hyemin, and Chi-Young Kim. The Things You Can See Only When You Slow down: How to Be Calm and Mindful in a Fast-Paced World. Penguin Books, 2017. "Demonstrations of love are small, compared to the great thing that is hidden behind them." - Khalil Gibran *The Prophet*

58. Gottman, John, PhD, and Julie Schwartz Gottman, PhD. "What Do Women Really Want?" In *The Man's Guide To Women*, 8-11. New York, NY: Rodale, 2016.

59. Eggerichs, Dr. Emerson. ""How to Spell C-H-A-I-R-S to Your Husband." In *Love & Respect: The Love She Most Desires; The Respect He Desperately Needs*, 193-528. Nashville, TN: Integrity Publishers, 2004.

60. Peterson, J. B. (2019, March 25). Psychological Significance of the Biblical Stories - Jordan B Peterson. Retrieved November 22, 2020, from https://www.jordanbpeterson.com/bible-series/ ; "...things that you regard as impossible will happen."

61. Liu, Yan, et al. "Social Bonding Decreases the Rewarding Properties of Amphetamine through a Dopamine D1 Receptor-Mediated Mechanism." The Journal of Neuroscience: the Official Journal

of the Society for Neuroscience, U.S. National Library of Medicine, 1 June 2011, www.ncbi.nlm. nih.gov/pubmed/21632917/.

62. Liu, Yan, et al. "Nucleus Accumbens Dopamine Mediates Amphetamine-Induced Impairment of Social Bonding in a Monogamous Rodent Species." Proceedings of the National Academy of Sciences of the United States of America, National Academy of Sciences, 19 Jan. 2010, www.ncbi.nlm. nih.gov/pubmed/20080553/.

63. Mylett, Ed, and Dr. Joe Dispenza. "Unlock The Unlimited Power of Your Mind Today! | Ed Mylett & Dr. Joe Dispenza." YouTube, 21 Mar. 2019, http://youtu.be/ereahWKwNV8. 48:10-48:24

64. Bauer, Viktor, and Ružena Sotníková. "Nitric Oxide--the Endothelium-Derived Relaxing Factor and Its Role in Endothelial Functions." General Physiology and Biophysics, U.S. National Library of Medicine, Dec. 2010, www.ncbi.nlm.nih.gov/ pubmed/21156995/.

65. Hostetler, Caroline M, and Andrey E Ryabinin. "Social Partners Prevent Alcohol Relapse Behavior in Prairie Voles." Psychoneuroendocrinology, U.S. National Library of Medicine, Jan. 2014, www.ncbi. nlm.nih.gov/pubmed/24275014/.

66. Patrick, Rhonda, and Matthew Walker. "Dr. Matthew Walker on Sleep for Enhancing Learning, Creativity, Immunity, and Glymphatic System." YouTube, FoundMyFitness, 28 Feb. 2019, http://

youtu.be/bEbtf7uS6P8. "Loneliness increases mortality rate by and upwards of 45%"

67.   Maslar, Dawn. "How Your Brain Falls In Love | Dawn Maslar | TEDxBocaRato." YouTube, TEDx, 5 July 2016,http:// youtu.be/eyq2Wo4eUDg.

Chapter 3| Models | Figures of Excellence

68.   Hadot, Pierre. What Is Ancient Philosophy? Harvard Univ. Press, 2004. Pg. 11,12,14,16,17

69.   Machiavelli, Niccolò, and Peter Constantine. The Prince. Arcturus, 2009. Pg. 70

70.   "Greg Plitt." Official Website of Greg Plitt, www. gregplitt.com/.

71.   Rose , Brian, and Grant Cardone. "Grant Cardone's Most Revealing Interview EVER with London Real." YouTube, 8 June 2018, youtu.be/ PujltB4VZlI.

72.   Cardone, Grant. How to Create Wealth Investing in Real Estate. Grant Cardone Training Technologies, 2018. Pg 4-5

73.   Keuilian, Bedros, and Ed Mylett. "Ed Mylett - An Inside Look | Empire Podcast Show." YouTube, 28 Feb. 2018 ,https://youtu.be/en3Qf4Fh9IA

74.   Forbes, Forbes Magazine, www.forbes.com/ lists/2008/10/billionaires08_Arthur-Williams-Jr_DA4B.html.

75.   "Gadsden Times." Google News Archive Search, Google, news.google.com/

newspapers?nid=1891&dat=19951107&id=Krw
fAAAAIBAJ&sjid=FNgEAAAAIBAJ&pg=4898,
678628.

76. Chicago Tribune. "BILLIONAIRE PAYS $70
MILLION TO SETTLE FALWELL'S DEBTS."
Chicagotribune.com, 30 Aug. 2018, www.chi-
cagotribune.com/news/ct-xpm-1998-02-03-
9802040368-story.html.

77. Williams, Arthur. "ART WILLIAMS JUST DO
IT SPEECH." YouTube, 7 May 2012, http://
youtu.be/7R9c0RAz678.

78. Whitworth, William, and William Whitworth.
"Kentucky-Fried." The New Yorker, The New
Yorker, 19 June 2017, www.newyorker.com/
magazine/1970/02/14/kentucky-fried.

79. Ozersky Josh. Colonel Sanders and the American
Dream. University of Texas press, 2017.

80. Darden, Bob. Secret Recipe: Why KFC Is Still
Cookin after 50 Years. Tapestry Press, 2002.

81. Smith, J. Y. "Col. Sanders, the Fried-Chicken
Gentleman, Dies." The Washington Post, WP
Company, 17 Dec. 1980, www.washingtonpost.
com/archive/local/1980/12/17/col-sanders-the-
fried-chicken-gentleman-dies/64925eb3-3a20-
4851-afbc-ba4fe16e9770/?noredirect=on&utm_
term=.99d8e7c4e818.

82. Feloni, Richard. "Tony Robbins Started out as a
Broke Janitor - Then He Saved a Week's Worth

of Pay, and the Way He Spent It Changed His Life." Google, Business Insider , 4 Oct. 2017, www. google.com/amp/s/amp.businessinsider.com/tony-robbins-changed-his-life-at-17-years-old-2017-10.

83.   Rohn , Jim. "Jim Rohn Best Life Ever." YouTube, 27 Dec. 2015, https://youtu.be/6ySBv-HHyK4

84.   Rohn, Jim. "Jim Rohn Personal Development Seminar." YouTube, 7 Feb. 2016, http://youtu.be/jnBdNkkceZw.

85.   Von, Theo, and Jocko Willink. "Jocko Willink on His Punk Band and Meeting Henry Rollins." YouTube, 11 Aug. 2018, http://youtu.be/wTuEm46tR6k.

86.   Young, Ed, and Marcus Luttrell. "Exclusive Interview - 'Lone Survivor' Navy Seal Marcus Luttrell w/ Ed Young." YouTube, 6 Aug. 2013, http://youtu.be/vcnyeIPyXG8.

87.   Luttrell, Marcus. "Marcus Luttrell 'Lone Survivor' Speech." YouTube, 9 Dec. 2014, http://youtu.be/H_Pi42Hv858.

88.   Luttrell, Marcus. "An Unstoppable Mind - MOST Powerful Motivation (The Lone Survivor) NAVY SEAL." YouTube, 14 Apr. 2018, https://youtu.be/8M0d-j7-Lk4.

89.   Schneiderman , R. M. "Why Mohammad Gulab, the Savior of Navy SEAL Marcus Luttrell, Claims 'Lone Survivor' Got It Wrong." Newsweek , Google , www.google.com/amp/s/www.newsweek.

com/2016/06/10/mohammad-gulab-marcus-luttrell-navy-seal-lone-survivor-operation-red-wings-458139.html?amp=1.

90. Donnelly, Tim. "9 Brilliant Inventions Made by Mistake." Inc.com, Inc., 15 Aug. 2012, www.inc.com/tim-donnelly/brilliant-failures/9-inventions-made-by-mistake.html.

91. Rilke, Rainer Maria. Letters to a Young Poet. Volume One, 1892-1910 Volume Two, 1910-1926, W. W Norton and Company Inc. Pg. 64 "greater confidence than our joys."

92. Machiavelli, Niccolò, and Peter Constantine. The Prince. Arcturus, 2009. Pg. 70

93. Britannica, The Editors of Encyclopaedia. "Philopoemen." Encyclopædia Britannica, Encyclopædia Britannica, Inc., 9 Apr. 2008, www.britannica.com/biography/Philopoemen.

94. Machowicz, Richard. "Indomitable Spirit - Motivational Video (HD)." YouTube, 15 Nov. 2014, https://youtu.be/z4XYkQdTTWE.

95. Willink , Jocko. "Extreme Ownership | Jocko Willink | TEDxUniversityofNevada." YouTube, 2 Feb. 2017, http://youtu.be/ljqra3BcqWM.

96. Trei, Lisa, and Lisa Trei. "New Study Yields Instructive Results on How Mindset Affects Learning." Stanford University, 7 Feb. 2007, news.stanford.edu/news/2007/february7/dweck-020707.html.

97. Voss, Christopher. "An FBI Negotiator's Secret to Winning Any Exchange | Inc." YouTube, 7 Jan. 2019, http://youtu.be/llctqNJr2IU.

98. Shapiro, Fred R. "Who Wrote the Serenity Prayer." The Chronicle of Higher Education, The Chronicle of Higher Education, 28 Apr. 2014, www.chronicle.com/article/Who-Wrote-the-Serenity-Prayer-/146159.

99. Clark, Derek, and Leonardo De Angelis. "A Story Of Greatness | Strive To Be Greatness | Motivational Video - Motivation For Life HD." YouTube, 9 Nov. 2014, http://youtu.be/mHkPB1b4wxQ.

100. Campbell, Barbara J. "Bone Health Basics - OrthoInfo - AAOS." OrthoInfo, May 2012, orthoinfo.aaos.org/en/staying-healthy/bone-health-basics/.

101. Ericsson, K. Anders, et al. The Role of Deliberate Practice in the Acquisition of Expert Performance. R. Th. Krampe, 1993. Pg. 369-370

102. Burchard, Brendon. High Performance Habits: How Extraordinary People Become That Way. Hay House, Inc., 2017. Chapter 3. "is a role model cheering you on."

103. Marden, Orison Swett, and G. R. Devitt. Success Library. Vol. 10, Success Co., 1901. Pg. 449. "Your memory is like a spirit."

104. Solženicyn, Aleksandr, and Thomas P. Whitney. The Gulag Archipelago. Harper & Row, 1975. "a piece of his own heart?"

105. Milo, Ron, and Ron Philips. "» How Quickly Do Different Cells in the Body Replace Themselves?" Cell Biology by the Numbers How Quickly Do Different Cells in the Body Replace Themselves Comments, book.bionumbers.org/how-quickly-do-different-cells-in-the-body-replace-themselves/.

Chapter 4 | On Influence

106. Divine, Mark, and Jordan Harbinger. "Jordan Harbinger on Building Social Capital Both Personally and Professionally." Unbeatable Mind, unbeatablemind.com/jordan-harbinger/?utm_campaign=jordan-harbinger&utm_medium=guest-social&utm_source=podcast-guest&utm_content=jordan-harbinger&utm_term=social-media-guest.

107. Coyle , Danial. Culture Code: The Secrets of Highly Successful Groups. Random House Business, 2019.

108. Steen, Duncan. "Meditations (Unabridged)." Naxos AudioBooks, 8 Dec. 2018, www.naxosaudiobooks.com/meditations-unabridged/.

109. Pease, Allan, and Barbara Pease. The Definitive Book of Body Language. Orion, 2006.

Chapter 5 | On Leadership

110. Peterson, Jordan. "Jordan Peterson Tells The Story Of Marduk." YouTube, 2 Oct. 2017, http://youtu.be/la6ROCNOGY8.

111. Mark, Joshua J. "Marduk." Ancient History Encyclopedia, Ancient History Encyclopedia, 7 May 2019, www.ancient.eu/Marduk/.

112. Peterson, Jordan. "Jordan Peterson - The Story of Marduk Part 2." YouTube, 15 May 2018, http://youtu.be/1AMtTBxmQb0.

113. Hadot, Pierre, and Michael Chase. What Is Ancient Philosophy? Belknap Press of Harvard Univ. Press, 2004. Pg. 11-12

114. Mazarakis, Anna. "Former Apple CEO John Sculley Is Working on a Startup That He Thinks Could Become Bigger than Apple." Business Insider, Business Insider, 10 Aug. 2017, www.businessinsider.com/john-sculley-interview-healthcare-pepsi-apple-steve-jobs-2017-8.

115. "'You Really Have No Choice but to Fight and to Win the Day.'" Stars and Stripes, www.stripes.com/news/special-reports/heroes/heroes-2015/you-really-have-no-choice-but-to-fight-and-to-win-the-day-1.349644. "Never above you, never below you, always beside you."

116. Greene, Robert. "Understand THIS... & You Won't Waste Anymore Time | Advice That Will Change Your Future." YouTube, 13 May 2019, https://youtu.be/4HZLAHFBBgM @ 5:30 on Negative Capability

117. Machiavelli, Niccolò. Modern New York Library. Translated by Peter Constantine, Modern Library, 2008. "It is man's nature to obligate himself as much for the benefits he gives as for the benefits he receives."

118. Machiavelli, Niccolò. Modern New York Library. Translated by Peter Constantine, Modern Library, 2008. Ch. 15, 18. Pg. 72, 81-83.

119. Mella, Aberto. "The Warrior in The Garden." The Gentlemen's Brotherhood, 30 Jan. 2017, www. thegentlemensbrotherhood.com/inspiration/ the-warrior-in-the-garden/.

120. Cardone, Grant. "Grant Cardone Closes - The Closer's Survival Guide." Grant Cardone Closes - The Closer's Survival Guide, closeorlose.info/. "Meaning of the word nice."

121. Washington. , George. "First Annual Address to Both Houses of Congress - Friday, January 08, 1790." George Washington's Mount Vernon, www. mountvernon.org/library/digitalhistory/quotes/ article/to-be-prepared-for-war-is-one-of-the-most-effectual-means-of-preserving-peace/.

122. Peterson, J. B. (2020, May 25). The Best Men I Know Are Dangerous. Retrieved May 25, 2020, from https://youtu.be/zSErYhxNLX0 "The best men I know are dangerous."

123. Willink, Jocko, et al. "Jocko Podcast 129 w/ Echo Charles: 'The General Principles of War', Frederick The Great." YouTube, 15 June 2018, http:// youtu.

be/qRBldwRsSRE. "The finest medallions have a reverse side." "Effectual means of preserving peace."

124. Watts, Alan. "Alan Watts - Outwitting the Devil." YouTube, 26 Nov. 2015, http://youtu.be/wAGdinXZjSc. "...but as a fervent cook, don't overdo it." @ 1:20-1:52.

125. Willink, Jocko, and Dave Hall. "Jocko Podcast 150 w/ Dave Hall and Josh Hall: Drafted to Vietnam, Surfing and Surfboards." YouTube, 7 Nov. 2018, http://youtu.be/kjF9uHZW_QE. @ 1:09:00-1:13:40

126. Trollope , Anthony. "Autobiography of Anthony Trollope." Www.24gamma. Com, Project Gutenberg Ebooks , 4 Oct. 2002, www.24grammata.com/wp-content/uploads/2011/12/Autobiography-of-Anthony-Trollope-24grammata.com .pdf. Pg. 39 "...spasmodic Hercules."

127. Rohn, Jim. "Jim Rohn Best Life Ever." YouTube, 27 Dec. 2015, https://youtu.be/6ySBv-HHyK4 "...Rest very little."

128. U.S. National Library of Medicine. (n.d.). *Norepinephrine*. National Center for Biotechnology Information. PubChem Compound Database. Retrieved October 30, 2021, from https://pubchem.ncbi.nlm.nih.gov/compound/Norepinephrine.

129. Crum, Alia J., et al. Stanford, 27 Aug. 2016, httrps://.stanford.edu/sites/g/files/sbiybj9941/f/

crumetal_mindsetthreatchallenge_8.27.16.pdf.
Pg. 18.

130. McGonigal, Kelly. "How to Make Stress Your
      Friend | Kelly McGonigal." YouTube, 4 Sept. 2013,
      http://youtu.be/RcGyVTAoXEU.

131. Sara, Susan J. "Locus Coeruleus in Time with
      the Making of Memories." Current Opinion in
      Neurobiology, Elsevier Current Trends, 2 Aug.
      2015, www.sciencedirect.com/science/article/abs/
      pii/S0959438815001129?via=ihub.

132. Berridge, Craig W, et al. "Noradrenergic
      Modulation of Wakefulness/Arousal." Sleep
      Medicine Reviews, U.S. National Library of
      Medicine, Apr. 2012, www.ncbi.nlm.nih.gov/pmc/
      articles/PMC3278579/.

133. Martin, R A, and J P Dobbin. "Sense of Humor,
      Hassles, and Immunoglobulin A: Evidence for a
      Stress-Moderating Effect of Humor." International
      Journal of Psychiatry in Medicine, U.S. National
      Library of Medicine, 1988, www.ncbi.nlm.nih.gov/
      pubmed/3170082/.

134. Martin, R A, and J P Dobbin. "Sense of Humor,
      Hassles, and Immunoglobulin A: Evidence for a
      Stress-Moderating Effect of Humor." International
      Journal of Psychiatry in Medicine, U.S. National
      Library of Medicine, 1988, www.ncbi.nlm.nih.gov/
      pubmed/3170082/.

135. Berk RA. The active ingredients in humor:
      psychophysiological benefits and risks

for older adults. Educational Gerontology. 2001;27(3-4):323–339.

136. Pease, Allan, et al. The Definitive Book of Body Language. PTS Publishing House, 2015. "Laughing Till You Cry" Pg. 82

137. Partners, Green Peak, and J. P. Flaum. "Research Results: Nice Guys Finish First When It Comes to Company Performance." GlobeNewswire News Room, "GlobeNewswire", 15 June 2010, www.globenewswire.com/ news-release/2010/06/15/1209139/0/en/ Research-Results-Nice-Guys-Finish-First-When-It-Comes-to-Company-Performance.html.

138. Bilyeu , Tom, and Jay Shetty. "How to Find Your Purpose | Jay Shetty on Impact Theory." YouTube, 20 Feb. 2018, http://youtu.be/GXoErccq0vw. "The Head, The Heart and The Hand."

139. Maxwell, John C. What Successful People Know about Leadership: Advice from Americas #1 Leadership Authority. Center Street, 2016. Pg. 108-109 "Heart, Hope, Hurt."

140. Willink, Jocko, et al. "Jocko Podcast 152 w/ Derek Herrera: Discipline, Drive, and Sacrifice. The Ethos of a Marine Raider." YouTube, 21 Nov. 2018, http://youtu.be/uvAlZ8YzPyY.

141. Rilke, Rainer Maria. Letters to a Young Poet. Volume One, 1892-1910 Volume Two, 1910-1926, W. W Norton and Company Inc. Pg. 72 "been able to find those words."

Chapter 6 | Gifts and Abilities

142. Rohn, Jim. "Jim Rohn Best Life Ever." YouTube, 27 Dec. 2015, https://youtu.be/6ySBv-HHyK4 "If you work on your gifts, they will make room for you". @ 4:21:16

143. Marston, Ama, and Stephanie Marston. Type R: Transformative Resilience for Thriving in a Turbulent World. PublicAffairs, 2018. "Our institutions and even our nations." Pg. 17

144. Page, Ken. Deeper Dating: How to Drop the Games of Seduction and Discover the Power of Intimacy. Shambhala Publications, 2015. "key to our deepest love and life-meaning."

145. Jung, C. G. The Archetypes and the Collective Unconscious. Princeton University Press, 1980. Pg. 127. Paragraph 228. ""Effort to obtain them ourselves."

146. Peterson, J. B. (2017, May 27). 2017 Maps of Meaning 12 Final: The Divinity of the Individual. Retrieved June 4, 2020, from https://youtu.be/6V1eMvGGcXQ "...an abstract of proper being." @ 1:50:58-1:51:24

Chapter 7 | Mastery

147. Suzuki, Shunryū, et al. Zen Mind, Beginner's Mind. Shambhala, 2011.

148. Saban, Nick, et al. How Good Do You Want to Be?: A Champion's Tips on How to Lead and Succeed at Work and in Life. Ballantine Books,

2007. "...The process is the price you pay for victory." Pg. 156

149. Gottman, John, et al. The Man's Guide to Women. Rodale, 2016.

150. Willink, Jocko. "Jocko Podcast 80 with Echo Charles - Musashi, 'The Book of Five Rings.'" YouTube, 21 June 2017, http://youtu.be/uq0Skb529q8.

151. Willink, Jocko, and Timothy Ferris. "Jocko Podcast 100 w/ Tim Ferriss - Musashi. Warrior Code and Life." YouTube, 16 Nov. 2017,http:// youtu.be/7GNRn3GtJ3g.

152. Mason, Stephen F. A History of the Sciences. Macmillan General Reference. Pg. 550

153. Greitens, Eric. Resilience: Hard-Won Wisdom for Living a Better Life. Mariner Books / Houghton Mifflin Harcourt, 2016. Pg. 46 "Mastery lives quietly atop a mountain of mistakes."

154. Rohn, Jim. "Jim Rohn: Ambition - How Desire Magnetizes Success Abundance Law Of Success." Youtube, 13 Nov. 2017, http://youtu.be/I4xDh5i-Al8. 13:25-15:45.

155. McKay, Kate. "Freedom From & Freedom To." The Art of Manliness, 7 Nov. 2018, www.artofmanliness.com/articles/freedom-from-freedom-to/.

156. Marden, Orison Swett, and G. R. Devitt. Success Library. Vol. 10, Success Co., 1901. Pg.498

"Transmuting Knowledge Into Power"."..power to the many."

157. Sarett, Lew, et al. Basic Principles of Speech. Houghton Mifflin, 1966. "..he is not whipped."

158. Cartwright, Mark. "Sisyphus." Ancient History Encyclopedia, Ancient History Encyclopedia, 14 Dec. 2016, www.ancient.eu/sisyphus/.

159. Itani, Mustapha. "Camus, Suicide, and Imagining Sisyphus Happy - Mustapha Itani." Medium, Medium, 12 Apr. 2019, medium.com/@ mustaphahitani/camus-suicide-and-imagining-sisyphus-happy-bec124dad750.

160. Carl Von. On War. Edited by Michael Howard and Peter Paret, Princeton University Press, 1976. Pg. 109 "... the mental gift that we call imagination."

161. "'If You Betray Me, Then I Have to See You Differently' Jordan Peterson - Grey's Model." YouTube, 9 May 2018, http://youtu.be/ FYUjo7zvz4A.

162. Peterson, Jordan B. "Your Conscience Is Always Telling You The Next Step - Jordan Peterson." YouTube, 17 July 2019, http://youtu.be/ WRKwNEI2nmo. 9:35-10:38

163. Bloom, Paul. "What We Miss." The New York Times, The New York Times, 4 June 2010, www. nytimes.com/2010/06/06/books/review/ Bloom-t.html.

164. Peterson, Jordan B. "2015 Personality Lecture 13: Existentialism: Nazi Germany and the USSR." YouTube, 26 Feb. 2015, https://youtu.be/XY7a1RXMbHI. 1:10:00-1:13:51.

Chapter 8 | Sabbath

165. "A Quote by Eleanor Brownn." Goodreads, Goodreads, www.goodreads.com/quotes/4295989-rest-and-self-care-are-so-important-when-you-take-time.

166. Lieberman, Matthew D. (University Of California Los Angeles, Matthew. Social - Why Our Brains Are Wired to Connect. Oxford University Press, 2015.

167. Levitin, Daniel J. The Organized Mind: Thinking Straight in the Age of Information Overload. Dutton, 2016.

168. Burchard, Brendon. High Performance Habits. Hay House, 2017.

169. Rohn, Jim. "How to Have the Best Year Ever! - Personal Development Life Coaching by Jim Rohn." YouTube, 22 Sept. 2017, http://youtu.be/6QVOBsS6ECY. 2:42:20

Chapter 9 | Friendship

170. Shenk, J. W. (2006). The Reign of Reason. In Lincoln's Melancholy How Depression Challenged a President and Fueled His Greatness (p. 103). New York, New York: Mariner Books. "...consists of his friendships."

171. Pattakos, Alex. The Meaning Of Friendship In A Social-Networked World. 7 Dec. 2017, www.huffpost.com/entry/the-meaning-of-friendship_b_761740. "...A single soul dwelling in two bodies."

172. Encyclopedia of Quotations A; Asking." Treasury of Thought. Forming an Encyclopædia of Quotations from Ancient and Modern Authors, by Maturin M. Ballou, Houghton, Mifflin, 1899, pp. 36–36. "...from the kitchen smells of smoke."

173. Washington, Geroge. "Founders Online: From George Washington to Bushrod Washington, 15 January 1783." National Archives and Records Administration. Accessed November 05, 2021. https://founders.archives.gov/documents/Washington/99-01-02-10429.

174. Peterson, Jordan B. "2017 Personality 15: Biology/Traits: The Limbic System." YouTube. March 13, 2017. Accessed November 05, 2021. https://youtu.be/AqkFg1pvNDw.

175. Peterson, Jordan B. "2017 Personality 16: Biology/Traits: Incentive Reward/Neuroticism." YouTube. March 13, 2017. Accessed November 05, 2021. https://youtu.be/ewU7Vb9ToXg

176. Peterson, Jordan B. "2017 Personality 17: Biology and Traits: Agreeableness." YouTube. March 29, 2017. Accessed November 05, 2021. https://youtu.be/G1eHJ9DdoEA.

177. Peterson, Jordan B. "2017 Personality 18: Biology & Traits: Openness/Intelligence/Creativity I." YouTube. April 18, 2017. Accessed November 05, 2021. https://youtu.be/D7Kn5p7TP_Y.

178. Peterson, Jordan B. "2017 Personality 19: Biology & Traits: Openness/Intelligence/Creativity II." YouTube. May 02, 2017. Accessed November 05, 2021. https://youtu.be/fjtBDa4aSGM.

179. Peterson, Jordan B. "2017 Personality 20: Biology & Traits: Orderliness/Disgust/Conscientiousness." YouTube. May 08, 2017. Accessed November 05, 2021. https://youtu.be/MBWyBdUYPgk.

Chapter 10 | On Death

180. Ganzales, Laurence. Deep Survival. W.W. Norton & Company, 2005. Pg. 294 " "Every year you pass an anniversary unaware: The anniversary of your own death."

181. Herodotus, and Robert Waterfield. Histories. Oxford University Press, 1998. Pg. 14-15

182. Marden, Orison Swett, and George Raywood Devitt. The Consolidated Library. Bureau of National Literature and Art, 1907. "What It Is To Be A Man"

183. Carnegie , Dale. How to Win Friends and Influence People. Simon & Schuster , 2009. Pg. 18 "until the end of his days."

184. Marden, Orison Swett, and George Raywood Devitt. The Consolidated Library. Bureau of National Literature and Art, 1907. "Reserve Corps"

185. Watts, A. (Trans.). (2020, June 23). *Alan Watts - Bhagavad Gita (remastered audio)*. YouTube. Retrieved October 30, 2021, from https://youtu.be/UeU3kE_66OQ. 4:32-5:26.

186. "Alan Watts - Sudden Enlightenment." YouTube, 17 Dec. 2015, https://youtu.be/LlAQaakSEzE. @ 15:47 - 16:09 "...it was hid so carefully."

187. Sarett, Lew, et al. Basic Principles of Speech. Houghton Mifflin, 1966. "Prodigal".

188. Marden, Orison Swett, and G. R. Devitt. Success Library. Vol. 10, Success Co., 1901. Pg. 457 "...a miser of minutes"

189. Seeger, Alan. "I Have a Rendezvous with Death by Alan Seeger." Poetry Foundation. Accessed November 05, 2021. https://www.poetryfoundation.org/poems/45077/i-have-a-rendezvous-with-death.

190. Marden, Orison Swett, and George Raywood Devitt. The Consolidated Library. Bureau of National Literature and Art, 1907. "What It Is To Be A Man."